W9-BHV-604

GENE-ENVIRONMENT INTERACTION IN COMMON DISEASES

GENE-ENVIRONMENT INTERACTION IN COMMON DISEASES

Proceedings of the Symposium on Gene-Environment Interaction in Common Diseases held February 11-12, 1976, Tokyo
Sponsored by the Japan Medical Research Foundation

Edited by
Eiji Inouye and Hideo Nishimura

UNIVERSITY PARK PRESS
Baltimore • London • Tokyo

UNIVERSITY PARK PRESS
Baltimore • London • Tokyo

Library of Congress Cataloging in Publication Data
Main entry under title:

Gene-environment interaction in common diseases.

(Publication—The Japan Medical Research Foundation; no. 2)
Papers presented at a symposium sponsored by the Japan Medical Research Foundation.
1. Medical genetics—Congresses. 2. Environmentally induced diseases—Congresses. 3. Human population genetics—Congresses. 4. Diseases—Animal models—Congresses.
I. Inouye, Eiji, 1919– II. Nishimura, Hideo, 1912–
III. Igaku Kenkyū Shinkō Zaidan. IV. Series: Igaku Kenkyū Shinkō Zaidan. Publication—The Japan Medical Research Foundation; no. 2.
RB155.G35 616′.042 77–3622
ISBN 0–8391–1116–9

© JAPAN MEDICAL RESEARCH FOUNDATION, 1977
UTP 3047–68571–5149

Printed in Japan

All rights reserved.

Originally published by
UNIVERSITY OF TOKYO PRESS

Foreword

The development of modern medicine has contributed to clarifying the etiology and treatment of various diseases as well as to improving public health and welfare. However, there are still many debilitating diseases of unknown etiology and without effective treatment. The Japan Medical Research Foundation was established in October 1973 in order to promote research on such diseases using funds from non-governmental sources.

It is well known that both genetic and environmental components are involved in the etiology of common diseases such as diabetes, essential hypertention, congenital heart diseases, cleft lip, and cleft palate. This first international symposium was held to exchange views on the etiology and pathogenesis of these common diseases, to look for new research tools, and to establish a firm basis for prevention and therapy of such diseases.

The Japan Medical Research Foundation is very pleased to support this symposium, and I am happy hopeful that the publication of its proceedings will make its work available to wide scientific readership.

February 20, 1977

Masayoshi Yamamoto
President
Japan Medical Research Foundation

Contents

Preface

In 1963 a group of scientists met at the World Health Organization and discussed the impact of genetic disorders on public health. According to the report prepared by the group (WHO, 1964), about 1 percent of live-born individuals have simple Mendelian disorders. The incidence of chromosome aberrations among the general population is at least 0.5 percent (see, for example, Jacobs *et al.*, 1970).

The above two categories, however, do not represent the entire spectrum of human genetic disorders. It is generally accepted that there is another category consisting of various common and familial disorders, the genetic predisposition to which is important in their etiology and symptom formation. According to the WHO report, developmental malformations affect 1.5 percent of the liveborn, and an additional 1 percent can be found at the age of 5 years. Constitutional, chronic, and degenerative disorders such as diabetes mellitus and idiopathic epilepsy constitute another 1 percent, and overall risk for live-born children is estimated to be at least 3.5 percent. If mental disorders such as schizophrenia and manic-depressive psychosis and primary (or subcultural) mental retardation are taken into account, where genetic predisposition is again considered to be important, the total risk may reach 6–7 percent.

Medical scientists and geneticists have scrutinized the pathogenesis of the first and second categories of genetic disorders. Measures of prevention have proved effective in treating some of these disorders. On the other hand, progress in research on disorders of the third category has been slow, mainly because of difficulties in analyzing the complex genetic mechanisms involved in their etiology and symptom formation.

Human geneticists and scientists of allied disciplines agree, however, that the time is ripe to exchange views on the genetic and environmental factors involved in the pathogenesis of common and familial disorders, from both theoretical and practical points of view. A committee was appointed by the Japan Medical Research Foundation, and a number of scientists interested in the topic were invited to participate in a two-day symposium. Among the proposed participants, only Prof. A. G. Motulsky, who was expected to deliver a paper and concluding remarks, could not attend.

All the papers and group discussions at the symposium were important and have served as valuable sources of information particularly relevant to future studies. However, some of the group discussions had to be omitted from this publication because of space limitations.

The editors wish to express sincere gratitude to the contributors to this volume and to all other participants to the symposium. Special thanks are due to the officers of the Japan Medical Research Foundation, who used their excellent skills in planning and carrying out the symposium. The editors are also greatly obliged to Ms. E. Hamao of the University of Tokyo Press.

REFERENCES

World Health Organization. 1964. Human Genetics and Public Health. WHO Technical Report Series No. 282.

Jacobs, P. A., Price, W. H., Law, P. (Eds). 1970. Human Population Cytogenetics, Pfizer Medical Monographs 5, Edinburgh University Press, Edinburgh.

The Editors

Introductory Remarks

Eiji Inouye

In the past, the most important human diseases were those which, like infectious diseases, are caused by exogenous factors. Thanks to the remarkable progress of preventive and therapeutic measures, the prevalence of such diseases has declined sharply in recent decades. Desire to improve the quality of life has also led people to accept planned parenthood, which has contributed greatly to a reduction in once high infant mortality rates.

Longer life spans have been achieved, and the human being, as a result, is more likely than before to suffer from non-exogenous diseases, which are less fatal but which can be chronic and which often result in costly disabilities.

Tuberculosis was once the most common cause of death in Japan. However, it has been replaced by cerebral apoplexia, cancer, and heart diseases as the most common causes of death since 1958. The annual death rate due to malignant neoplasms has apparently been increasing since 1947, not only among the over-60 age group, but also among those under 30 (Koizumi, 1971). Deaths among infants under one year of age were 60 per thousand in 1950, but dropped dramatically to 13 per thousand 20 years later.

The vast changes in categories and in the prevalence of diseases among humans has attracted the serious attention of medical practitioners, paramedical personnel, scientists, and officials engaged in public health administration and research, at both national and international levels. Diseases which had been less thoroughly investigated and were difficult to cure became the subjects of intensive and extensive study. To promote such research, the Japan Medical Research Foundation was established in 1974. The present symposium has been planned in order to disseminate information about current research on common diseases which still pose threats to public health.

We use the term "common diseases" to describe the subject of the present symposium. This term may sound curious and require further explanation. Many diseases are caused by single abnormal genes. Inborn errors of metabolism are examples. Such diseases are usually very rare, and their frequency in the general population is one in a hundred thousand or so. According to the classical theory of population genetics, this frequency represents a stabilized state, in which the rate of mutation and the rate of natural selection are of the same magnitude. In other words, any increase of an abnormal gene due to naturally occurring mutation is counterbalanced by a decrease due to natural selection operating on the affected individuals, thus maintaining a certain low level of frequency of the disease among the general population.

In contrast to these rare diseases caused by single abnormal genes, we are confronted with more common diseases with a frequency of one in a thousand or so. To cite a few examples, morbid risk of schizophrenia in the general population is between 8 and 9 per thousand in Europe and in Japan, if corrected for age. This figure is around one hundred times the risk of inborn errors of metabolism. Approximately the same frequency is seen in diabetes mellitus. The prevalence rate is between 15 and 23 per thousand among individuals aged over 60 years, according to a study conducted in Edinburgh (Smith *et al.*, 1972). Similarly, the frequency of central nervous system malformations is 6.2 per thousand, according to another survey conducted in Britain (Butler and Alberman, 1969). For all categories of major congenital malformations except Down's syndrome, a frequency of 23 per thousand was indicated in this survey.

The intensity of natural selection operating on individuals suffering from one of the above diseases may vary, but it is difficult to conceive such a high frequency due solely to an equilibrium between mutation and natural selection against single abnormal genes.

Numerous past studies on the above and other common diseases have indicated that the frequency of the diseases among near relatives of affected individuals is higher than that in the general population. The influence of the common environment shared by near relatives is often cited as a possible explanation for this family aggregation. If this were the case, the most profound effect would be observed among twins living together. In fact, however, it has been repeatedly indicated that the frequencies of such common diseases among monozygotic twin partners are higher than those among dizygotic twin partners. If we select investigations of common diseases and syndromes (including infectious diseases) from the literature, where at least three systematic twin studies have been conducted independently, the median frequencies are higher in monozygotic than in dizygotic twin partners, without a single exception. This result strongly indicates the presence of genetic predisposition in these common diseases. At the same time, we must not overlook the crucial importance of certain environmental factors, as is indicated by the presence of non-affected monozygotic twin partners and by the finding of apparent exogenous factors which might have caused the disease in monozygotic twin index cases.

Partly due to environmental factors in the etiology, most of the common and familial diseases do not show simple Mendelian segregation. Accumulated evidence indicates that genes at a number of loci are involved in these diseases. In some cases, the overall effect of the genes at many loci seems to be responsible for the genetic predisposition of an individual. In other cases, genes at different loci are responsible for respective entities, but the phenotypes are similar among them, so that a number of different genetic entities are included within a clinical entity. Other entities mainly caused by environmental factors may also be included in the clinical entity.

Analysis of such complex genetic mechanisms is not easy, but we are now beginning to have powerful tools which can be applied to a variety of diseases affecting different organ systems.

A few words about the term "interaction" between gene and environment. If we deal with both genes and environment, the two components are not necessarily independent. A certain genotype determines a phenotype only in the presence of a specific environment, while other genotypes do not. A classical example is the abnormal gene on the locus of glucose-6-phosphate-dehydrogenase and the intake of the antimalarial drug primaquine; the presence of both manifests hemolytic disorders. Where multiple loci are involved, this sort of gene-environment interaction should be borne in mind.

It is a source of particular satisfaction to me that experts on the above topics gathered for the present symposium. Exchanging views among the discipines of medicine, biology, and the allied sciences will certainly provide a firm basis for conducting further research and improving future human welfare.

REFERENCES

Bulter, N. R., and Alberman, E. D. 1969. *Perinatal problems: The second report of the 1958 British perinatal mortality survey*. Churchill Livingstone, Edinburgh, Scotland.

Koizumi, A. 1971. *Ningen seizon no seitaigaku* (Ecology of human survival). Kyorin Shoin, Tokyo, Japan.

Smith, C., Falconer, D. C., and Duncan, L. J. P. 1972. A statistical and genetic study of diabetes. II. Heritability of liability. *Ann. Hum. Genet.* **35**: 281–299.

I EPIDEMIOLOGY AND POPULATION GENETICS OF COMMON DISEASES

The Use of Registers in Morbidity Studies in Human Populations: Present and Future

James R. Miller

A register is a tool. In itself it cannot provide answers to the complexities of the question of gene-environment interaction in common diseases. However, a well-operated register can provide the mechanism by which some of the complexities can be approached.

In the minds of many people concerned with population aspects of disease, a register is a panacea: the establishment of a register will, in some mysterious way, resolve hitherto unresolvable problems. Such a view is naive in the extreme and has resulted in the failure of registers in the past. Registers can achieve only what they are designed to achieve, and many have failed because their goals were inadequately defined or because their expectations were incompatible with their designs. A properly designed register with clearly defined goals and case-finding procedures compatible with these goals can be useful in morbidity studies of genetically determined disease.

It is not my intent to review registers in detail. They may take many forms, may be large or small, and may deal with one disease (or a group of similar diseases) or encompass many diseases (for reviews see Miller and Lowry, 1976; Weddell, 1973). Disease registers have been used for the study of the epidemiology of diseases, for surveillance of health problems, for evaluation of treatment, for planning and evaluating services, and for research and education in a variety of health problems. Regardless of the format and goal(s), a good register is characterized by sound methods of ascertainment, proper follow-up of cases, and statistical and other utilization of the data.

Twin registers are often cited as examples of a form of register that is useful in determining the role of gene-environment interaction in chronic

Department of Medical Genetics, University of British Columbia, and Genetic Consultant, British Columbia Health Surveillance Registry.

diseases. Although twin registers have been used in several countries, in general the results have never measured up to the enthusiasm with which the registers were planned. The problem of obtaining unbiased samples of the various twin types, the need for large samples of twins to obtain even modest samples of a specific disease, and the difficulties of maintaining the long-term follow-up necessary in the study of chronic disease have resulted in a general skepticism about the practical value of such registers. Nevertheless, it is probably fair to say that many twin registers were improperly designed, and such failures should not deter those who are prepared to make the necessary efforts to design and operate such registers properly in the future.

In this presentation I should like to discuss three topics that will illustrate some of the uses of a register in morbidity studies of genetically determined disease: the determination of incidence and prevalence rates; cluster detection; and the determination of the natural history of specific diseases, using examples taken primarily from the British Columbia Health Surveillance Registry. The history and operation of this Registry have been described previously by Lowry *et al.* (1975). It has been in operation for over 20 years and comprises several registers concerned primarily with chronic handicapping disorders, including those that are genetically determined.

Incidence and Prevalence Rates

One of the most fundamental questions about a disease relates to the rate with which it enters a population (incidence) and occurs in a population at a particular time (prevalence). The incidence and prevalence rates of most genetically determined disease are unknown for most human populations, and no formal mechanisms exist for deriving estimates of these rates. A register in itself will not guarantee reliable rates, but it should provide the mechanisms for determining reasonable estimates of such rates.

Several years ago, it was estimated that close to two-thirds of the cases with a known etiology on the British Columbia Registry were, wholly or in part, genetically determined. Trimble and Doughty (1974) studied this load of disease in more detail, and from it they estimated that a minimum of 10 percent of newborns in B.C. would at some time in their lives exhibit a genetically determined handicap. This overall estimate and the estimates of the individual components of it have been criticized (particularly the underestimation of late-onset dominant disorders), but there is no question that the largest contribution to this genetic load derives from those diseases that involve complex gene-environment interactions.

Accurate determination of incidence and prevalence rates for specific diseases depends on two fundamental processes—classification and enumeration. In an age of molecular biology, it often comes as a shock to realize that most health jurisdictions cannot provide statistics on disease frequency because those in charge of such jurisdictions can neither classify nor count. To some extent, there is an excuse for the former deficiency, because no totally satisfactory classification of diseases exist. This simply reflects the complexities of human biology and the disease processes that affect it. However, a failure to count accurately is more difficult to comprehend.

The British Columbia Registry attempts to deal with both of these problems by using multiple sources of ascertainment with no upper age limit on case finding. This guarantees reliable numerators for incidence and prevalence fractions. The reliability of equally important demoninators is guaranteed by the fact that the Registry is part of the Provincial Division of Vital Statistics. Even with such guarantees, there are many problems associated with the derivation of such rates for single gene defects, let alone for more etiologically complex diseases.

Changes in incidence and prevalence rates are important. Lowry and his colleagues (1976) have recently looked for changes in rates for Down's syndrome (D.S.). They were intrigued by that fact that, although the proportion of women over 35 years of age among all those giving birth had declined dramatically, the crude incidence rate appeared to remain the same. Using records of cases of D.S. on the register linked to their birth registrations to derive maternal age, Lowry *et al.* derived crude incidence and age-specific rates for the period 1952–73. Over this period mean maternal age for both normal children and those with D.S. declined; the decline for all live births was from 27.4 to 25.0 years, and for cases of D.S. it was 34.1 to 28.8 years. At the beginning of this period, 54 percent of D.S. cases were born to women over 35 years of age, but by 1972 only 20 percent of cases were born to such women. This trend has been observed elsewhere, and there is no reason to suspect that it will alter. Despite this change in the maternal age pattern, the crude incidence rate for D.S. (mean 1.28/1,000 live births) has remained relatively constant over the 20-year period, except for 1969, when a statistically significant increase occurred. The significance of these findings is discussed by Lowry *et al.* My purpose in outlining them here is to make two points. First, the availability of the register data and their linkability to vital records made this extensive study possible and will make possible the continued monitoring of maternal age trends. Second, because most jurisdictional units lack the means of routinely deriving incidence and prevalence rates, we may be missing changes that have profound biological significance. One of the significant facts about D.S. was its association with advanced maternal age. If the trend recorded by Lowry and his colleagues continues (accompanied by the availability of amniocentesis), then this particular association will disappear. The fascinating fact that the age-adjusted rate may be increasing may pose more biological challenges about this intriguing disease.

Cluster Analysis

A clustering of a disease in time and space is usually evidence of the operation of non-genetic factors. Infectious diseases are excellent examples of clustering. The formal analysis of clusters of a chronic disease with a low frequency of occurrence is complex. It is often difficult to prove statistically that a suspected cluster is real, while in other circumstances it is often difficult to determine precisely what has caused a statistically proven cluster. Clusters of genetically determined diseases may reflect the presence of a mutagenic agent in the environment or of specific breeding isolates within a larger genetically heterogeneous population.

There are examples in several countries of registers or surveillance systems detecting clusters of congenital malformations (Miller and Lowry, 1976). Although some of these were attributable to changes in ascertainment and reporting, several have represented genuine biological phenomena; none, however, has yielded to detailed analysis in the sense of a teratogen being detected. However, the reassuring point is that these registers and/or monitoring systems in different countries, using quite diffeernt methods of statistical analysis, have successfully detected clusters. Recently Hook *et al.* (1976) have demonstrated ways in which the data collected in a multicenter registry system can be used to carry out cluster analysis (in this case, seasonal variation) on chromosomal aberrations.

I should like to extend the usual concept of cluster analysis discussed above to the occurrence of disease in specific high-risk genotypic groups. This type of study is difficult using a register unless there is access to additional information through some from of linkage system. The question whether specific subgroups in a population are at greater risk of developing a disease is not limited to genetically determined disabilities. The concept of the newborn risk register is an attempt to answer such a question. Such registers ascertained and followed up newborns judged to be at risk of developing problems because of adverse genetic, prenatal, obstetrical, and perinatal influences. Such registers were popular, particularly in Great Britain, 10 years ago. However, they have now fallen into disfavor because of a failure to exercise discrimination in ascertainment. Such registers were flooded with so many low-risk infants that the aims of the register were defeated. This is a salutory experience, but I don't believe that this failure should end attempts to use this concept. In British Columbia, we have only limited experience with risk registers, although one now exists in the Registry on children who were subjected to second trimester amniocentesis. Recently, the Registry has received a proposal to develop a stroke register, which includes the concept of a risk register in the form of a hypertension register. The aim, of course, is to determine what type of patients move from the risk register (hypertension) to the handicap register (stroke). This proposal is still in the formative stages, and it is obvious that the same problems which bedeviled the newborn risk registers could arise: the hypertension register could be swamped. However, I find the concept intriguing and hope it can be established in some form.

Attempts to delineate specific subpopulations of human beings who are at increased risk of developing disease because of genetic or other factors would be improved if more serious attention were given to the potential of record linkage (Acheson, 1967; Newcombe, 1967). Two of the keys to the success of a register are multiple sources of ascertainment, which provide a constant check on the completeness and accuracy of incoming information, and simplicity in the record on any one individual. This latter point is important but is frequently misunderstood. A register should not try to compile a complete, detailed file on every case. Rather, it should attempt to maintain a minimum of accurate diagnostic and identifying data, to enable the files to serve as a reliable index of cases that can be followed up. Follow-up activities may include direct contact, if necessary, but most frequently will involve consultation of health and vital records. It is for this reason that the integration of a register into a system of linked files is important. The fact that the British Columbia Registry is part of the Provincial Division of Vital Statistics made the study of Lowry *et al.* (1976) on D.S. possible. Newcombe (1967) has demonstrated his record linkage procedure using data from the British Columbia system.

Natural History

A well-operated register should provide mechanisms for obtaining an overview of the natural history of a disease by the development of appropriate follow-up studies and by provision of a reliable index of cases for special studies. The British Columbia Registry has served as the basis for several such projects. Miller and Gallagher (1975) have published the results of a follow-up study involving two age group cohorts comprising 13,100 individuals. The follow-up was successful in locating over 80 percent of cases and has demonstrated the load of residual handicap and the type of schooling required by a cohort of handicapped children. Gray and her colleagues (1972) used the Registry caseload for studies on Legg-Perthes disease and were able to demonstrate sound evidence for polygenic inheritance. The study of Lowry *et al.* (1976) on the changing maternal age pattern in D.S. used the register as an index.

Problems

There are many problems associated with the establishment and maintenance of a register. Most of these are of a routine nature, and it would be inappropriate to discuss them here (see Miller and Lowry, 1976). However, two points merit comment: the importance of defining the goals of a register and of constantly monitoring the intake and output to ensure that they are compatible with the goals cannot be overstressed. It is too easy to collect large volumes of information without monitoring its quality or usefulness. And, as Weddell (1973) has pointed out, computers make the collection of such data deceptively simple. In April 1975, an international group recommended that an international chromosome register *not* be established at this time (Hamerton, 1975). This decision was based upon a review of: the specific criteria for a register; what was expected of this particular register; and the analysis of a specific problem which might be resolved by the formation of such a register. This exercise is an ideal model of the steps to be followed before a decision is made to establish a register.

The question of security of confidential records is of concern to anyone responsible for the maintenance of large systems of data. The problem is not great if the only purpose of the system is to produce statistical data. However, if a register is to function as an index of cases for a variety of studies involving follow-up, then problems may develop. If the register is small, with limited access, these problems are minimal, but if the register is large and provides a base for many studies, then strict rules are essential. The British Columbia Registry operates under very strict rules which have been described elsewhere (Lowry *et al.*, 1975). Genetic registers of the type described by Emery and his colleagues (Emery *et al.*, 1974; Emery, 1976) and chromosome registers developing in the U.S.A. and elsewhere (Hecht, 1976) often include information on normal relatives who, while not affected with a disease, are at risk of developing the disease or of producing affected offspring. The registration of such individuals may be important in preventive counselling programs (as in Emery's RAPID system) or in determining the factors that may precipitate a late-onset disease. However, this type of registration may produce problems of overload and ethical issues unless there is a clear understanding of why such normal individuals are on the register.

Conclusion

The problems of analyzing gene-environment interaction in common diseases are some of the most important, but most difficult, in human medicine. As I said at the outset, a register cannot solve these problems directly but is only one tool in the unraveling of the complexities involved. Nevertheless, I believe a well-operated register is an important tool in this task, despite the real difficulties that have to be faced in establishing and maintaining such a system. I hope some of the examples I have given will convince you of my thesis.

REFERENCES

Acheson, E. D. (Ed.) 1967. *Record linkage in medicine*. E. and S. Livingstone, Edinburgh, Scotland.

Emery, A. E. H. 1976. A genetic register system for the ascertainment and prevention of inherited disease. *In* Emery, A. E. H., and Miller, J. R., *Registers for the detection and prevention of genetic disease*. Symposia Specialists, Miami, U.S.A.

Emery, A. E. H., Elliott, D., Moores, M., and Smith, C. 1974. A genetic register system (RAPID). *J. Med. Genet.* **11**: 145–151.

Gray, I. M., Lowry, R. B. and Renwick, D. G. H. 1972. Incidence and genetics of Legg-Perthes disease (Osteochondritis deformans) in British Columbia: Evidence of polygenic determination. *J. Med. Genet.* **9**: 197–202.

Hamerton, J. L. 1975. Human cytogenetic registries. *Humangenetik*. **29**: 177–181.

Hecht, F. 1976. Problems in the development of chromosome registers. *In* Emery, A. E. H., and Miller, J. R., *Registers for the detection and prevention of genetic disease*. Symposia Specialists, Miami, U.S.A.

Hook, E. B., Hoff, M. B., and Porter, I. H. 1976. A search for seasonal variation in trisomy 21 incidence in 1969–1973 in reports to a chromosome registry. (submitted to *Amer. J. Hum. Genet.*)

Lowry, R. B., Jones, D. C., Renwick, D. H. G., and Trimble, B. D. 1976. Down's syndrome in British Columbia, 1952–1973: Incidence and mean maternal age. *Teratology* **14**: 29–34.

Lowry, R. B., Miller, J. R., Scott, A. E., and Renwick, D. H. G. 1975. The British Columbia Registry for Handicapped Children and Adults: Evolutionary changes over 20 years. *Can J. Publ. Hlth.* **66**: 322–326.

Miller, J. R., and Gallagher, R. P. 1975. The use of a registry caseload survey in predicting trends in rehabilitative needs for the handicapped. *J. Med. Defic. Res.* **19**: 101–106.

Miller, J. R., and Lowry, R. B. 1976. Birth defects registries and surveillance. *In* Wilson J. G., and Fraser, F. C., *Handbook of teratology*. Plenum Press: New York, U.S.A. (in preparation).

Newcombe, H. B. 1967. Present state and long-term objective of the British Columbiap opulation study. Proc. 3rd Int. Congr. Hum. Genet. The Johns Hopkins Press, Baltimore, U.S.A.

Trimble, B. K., and Doughty, J. H. 1974. The amount of hereditary disease in human populations. *Ann. Hum. Genet.* **38**: 199–223.

Weddell, J. M. 1973. Registers and registries: a review. *Int. J. Epidemiol.* **2**: 221–228.

DISCUSSION 1

Epidemiologic Study of Stroke in Japanese Men Living in Japan, Hawaii and California: Prevalence of Stroke

Yo Takeya,[*1] *Hiroo Kato,*[*2] *Abraham Kagan,*[*3] *Jordan Popper,*[*3] *George G. Rhoads,*[*3] *G. Browne Goode,*[*4] *and Michael Marmot*[*5]

It is well known that the most prevalent killer in Japan is cerebrovascular disease, and storke mortality in Japan has been reported to be one of the highest in the world. Many Japanese people migrated to the United States, Hawaii, California, and so on. Among Japanese migrants and their offspring in the United States, stroke mortality is lower than it is in Japan.

In oreder to investigate the difference in the frequency of stroke between indigenous and migrant Japanese, an epidemiologic study of stroke in Japanese men living in Japan, Hawaii, and California was initiated in 1965. This tripartite collaborative study was nicknamed the "NI-HON-SAN Study." NI stands for Nippon (Japan in Japanese), HON means Honolulu in Hawaii, and SAN reflects San Francisco in California.

Cohorts of older and middle-aged men in Hiroshima and Nagasaki, Japan, in Honolulu, Hawaii, and in the eight counties of the San Francisco Bay Area of California participated in a series of examinations which were designed to be comparable in a number of important respects. In 1972, I joined the NI-HON-SAN Study as a clinical neurologist from Japan.

Here, I would like to present a quantitative assessment of the difference in stroke prevalence between the Japan and United States cohorts.

A detailed description of the recruitment of these study populations has been reported elsewhere. The Japan cohort consisted of 1,458 men participating in the adult health study program in Hiroshima and Nagasaki run by the Radiation Effects Research Foundation (formerly the Atomic Bomb

---

[*1] Health Center, Kyushu University, Fukuoka, Japan.

[*2] Radiation Effects Research Foundation, Hijiyama Park, Hiroshima, Japan.

[*3] Honolulu Heart Study, National Heart and Lung Institute, National Institute of Health, Honolulu, Hawaii, U.S.A.

[*4] Department of Medicine, The Permanente Medical Group, San Francisco, California, U.S.A.

[*5] Japanese-American Health Research, Division of Epidemiology, School of Public Health, University of California, Berkeley, California, U.S.A.

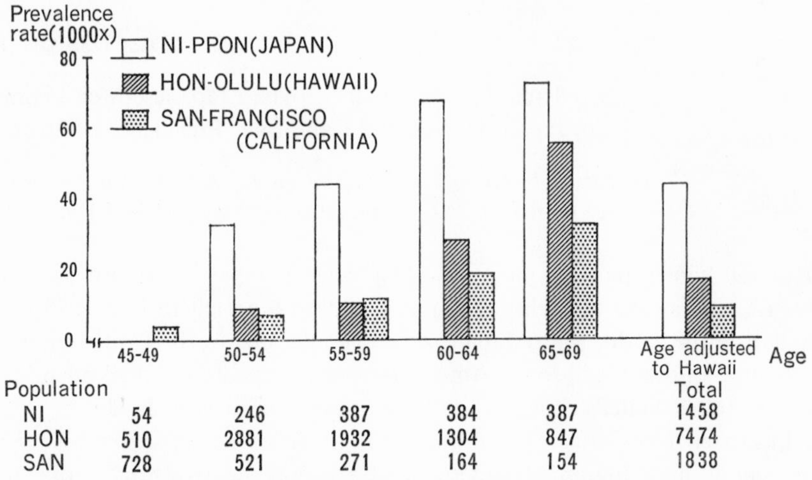

Population	45-49	50-54	55-59	60-64	65-69	Total
NI	54	246	387	384	387	1458
HON	510	2881	1932	1304	847	7474
SAN	728	521	271	164	154	1838

FIG. 1. Age-specific prevalence of history of stroke by study site.

Casualty Commission). These 1,458 men, aged 45–69 years, received examinations between 1972 and 1974.

Nearly half of the immigrants to Hawaii came from Hiroshima and Yamaguchi Prefectures at the southwestern tip of the main island of Honshu. The cohort in Hawaii consisted of 7,474 men of Japanese ancestry, aged 47–69 years, who participated in the second examination (1967–1970) of the Honolulu Heart Study.

Nearly half of the immigrants to California came from Hiroshima, Yamaguchi, and Fukuoka Prefectures. The California sample consisted of 1,838 men in the age group of 45–69 years, who were examined in 1969–1970.

In each of the three study sites, the subjects were asked the question, "Have you ever had a stroke?" An affirmative answer to this question constitutes one definition of stroke. The prevalence of such a history increases with age in each location. Under the age of 50, only three persons in California gave a history of a stroke. Because of the lower prevalence and the small number of men under the age of 50, a comparison in such younger men is inconclusive. A substantially higher frequency of stroke history was found in Japan than in the United States cohorts in each of the other four age groups.

The overall rates, age-adjusted by direct method to the age structure of the Hawaii cohort, are 43.9 in Japan, 17.3 in Hawaii, and 13.0 in California. That is, the age-adjusted rate in Japan is 2.5 times higher than in Hawaii and more than 3 times the rate in California.

The Honolulu neurologist met with the neurologists from Japan and California to set criteria for the definitive diagnosis of stroke. The participating neurologists in Japan and Hawaii met on three occasions to discuss case definition, and summary records of cases in the two sites were interchanged to provide a rough test of comparability. Twenty-six records were interchanged. Twenty-one were classified identically by two neurologists on a three-point scale of no stroke, possible stroke, and definite or probable stroke. If definite, probable, and possible strokes were combined, 25 diagnoses out of 26 (that is, 96.2%) were agreed on by two neurologists. This kind of interaction did not take place with the California neurologist.

Figure 2 shows the prevalence of stroke by 5-year age groups in the

TABLE 1. Comparison of stroke diagnosis of 26 cases.

		HAWAII		
		Definite & Probable	Possible	No Stroke
	Definite & Probable	13	1	
Japan	Possible	3	1	
	No Stroke		1	7

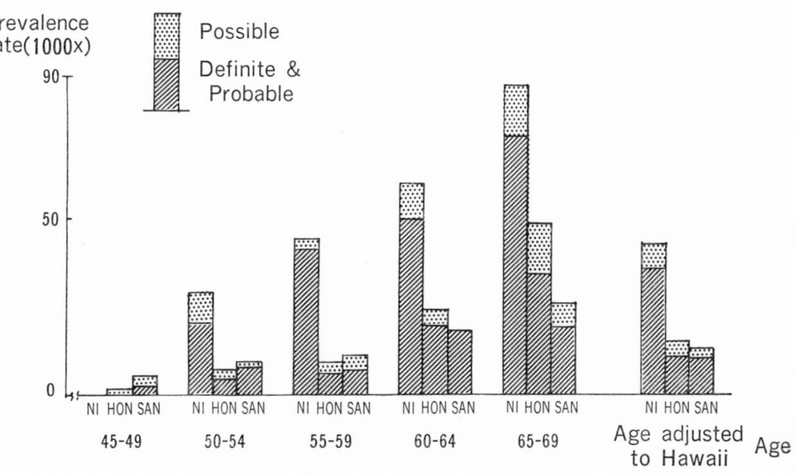

FIG. 2. Prevalence of stroke in examined Cohorts as determined by neurologist.

three sites as judged by the neurologist, his examination being supplemented if necessary by other available data. The striking excess frequency noted for Japan in Fig. 1 is again seen, whether one accepts only the definite and probable cases or includes the possible strokes as well. The age-adjusted prevalence of stroke (including possible cases) is calculated as 42.5, 15.0, and 13.0 in Japan, Hawaii, and California, respectively.

Two prevalence rates using two methods—one by history of stroke, the other by neurologist's judgment—are strikingly close. Although in interpreting the result of this study there remains the possible effect of non-response in the three cohorts, it seems likely that the prevalence of stroke in Japan is higher than in the United States cohorts.

My field is not epidemiology or genetics. As I am a clinical neurologist, I will not make any conclusive statement based on these data. This study, however, compares stroke prevalence in three population groups sharing a similar ethnic background but differing in geographic location and socio-cultural settings. The subjects are all Japanese males. The major Japanese site, Hiroshima, was the source of a large percentage of the Japanese migrants to Honolulu and the San Francisco Bay Area. Therefore, differences in stroke prevalence are likely to be indications of differing effects on the cerebrovascular system caused by differences in diet, life style, and environment.

REFERENCE

Kagan, A., *et al.* (1974): Epidemiologic studies of coronary heart disease and stroke in Japanese men living in Japan, Hawaii and California: demographic, physical, dietary and biochemical characteristics. *J. Chron. Dis.* **27**: 345–364.

DISCUSSION 2

Epidemiological Study with Early Human Prenatal Population

Hideo Nishimura

We have collected approximately 30,000 embryonic specimens that are obtained from legally conducted induced abortions. Each specimen is accompanied by the record of general and obstetric history. Undoubtedly such materials are useful for the study of pathogenesis of human malformations. Using this collection for epidemiological study is justified, since these materials can be regarded as a sample that represents adequately the total early prenatal population on the basis of the following facts: (1) unwanted pregnancy is fairly common and the operation of induced abortion is conducted without cumbersome procedures; (2) various parental variables such as parental age, parity, socioeconomic rank, etc., are not strikingly different from those in overall deliveries; (3) availability of useful specimens is dependent on chance, not on existence of malformations; and (4) obstetricians do not examine obtained early conceptuses before providing them to us.

Therefore, it is expected that studying this collection might furnish some new information not available from perinatal epidemiological study. In fact, the prevalence of polydactyly (hand) in embryos was found to be far higher than that in newborns (as shown in Table 1), and such a tendency is also found for various other malformations. This means that the study can reveal a wide range of maldevelopments thus hidden. Hence it is presumed

TABLE 1. Prevalence of polydactyly (hand).

	Embryos at stage 17–23 from induced abortion		
	Healthy mothers	Threatened abortion	Newborns*
Total no.	1,606	293	144,670
Pd (hand)	17 (1.06)	5 (1.71)	135 (0.09)

* Cited from Mitani, S. and Kitamura, Y., *Sanfujinka-Chiryo* (*Obstet. gynec. Ther.*) **17:** 265, 1968.

Department of Anatomy, Faculty of Medicine, Kyoto University, Kyoto, Japan.

that correlation study with such a population can provide us with more accurate information on the role of genetic and early prenatal environmental factors.

In view of this point, we are now in the process of transcribing our records, which are filled in by the obstetricians onto computer cards. When a sufficient number of cases are available, some useful conclusions will be drawn from the analysis. Moreover, considering that abortion laws are tending to become more liberal around the world, we are investigating the practicability of using the abortuses for malformation monitoring.

Some Aspects of the Genetic Epidemiology of Common Diseases*

N. E. Morton

The concept of host factors in disease is as old as medicine, but systematic study began only when public health measures had reduced the impact of infectious disease in industrial societies. Neel and Schull (1954) were apparently the first to recognize a new discipline of "epidemiological genetics" concerned with the interaction of heredity and disease. During the next decade Blumberg (1961) edited "Genetic polymorphisms and geographic variations in disease" and Neel, Shaw, and Schull (1965) produced "Genetics and the epidemiology of chronic diseases," in which Thomas Francis remarked:

> So when the human geneticist turns to disease and disorder in the population as his basis of genetic analysis, he is promptly in epidemiology. And where he asserts the concept of multiple factors to produce an effect, he is in fully cry epidemiologically. Conversely, where the epidemiologist seeks explanation for familial or other group aggregations of health or disease, he is immediately involved in genetic problems.

By 1967, when Morton, Chung, and Mi discussed problems in genetic epidemiology, there was general agreement that synthesis of goals and methods from epidemiology and genetics was inevitable and desirable. We preferred the term "genetic epidemiology" because determinants of familial aggregation may be purely environmental, whereas epidemiological genetics suggests an inappropriate prejudice against environmental hypotheses. A formal definition is:

Population Genetics Laboratory, University of Hawaii, Honolulu, U.S.A.

* This work was supported by Grant GM 17173 from the U.S. National Institutes of Health.

genetic epidemiology: a science that deals with the etiology, distribution, and control of disease in groups of relatives or with genetic causes of disease in populations.

"Genetic" is here used in a broad sense, to include both biological and cultural inheritance. The set of relatives may be as close as twins or as extended as an ethnic group.

Family Resemblance

The central problem in genetic epidemiology is to delineate family resemblance. Two complementary approaches have been used: *path analysis* of the correlations between relatives and indices of family environment or racial ancestry, and *segregation analysis* of patterns in nuclear families or larger pedigrees. These methods have different objectives and limitations (Morton, 1974, 1975a).

Path analysis is a special case of structural equations, which differ from more familiar multivariate systems in that measurement errors are permitted

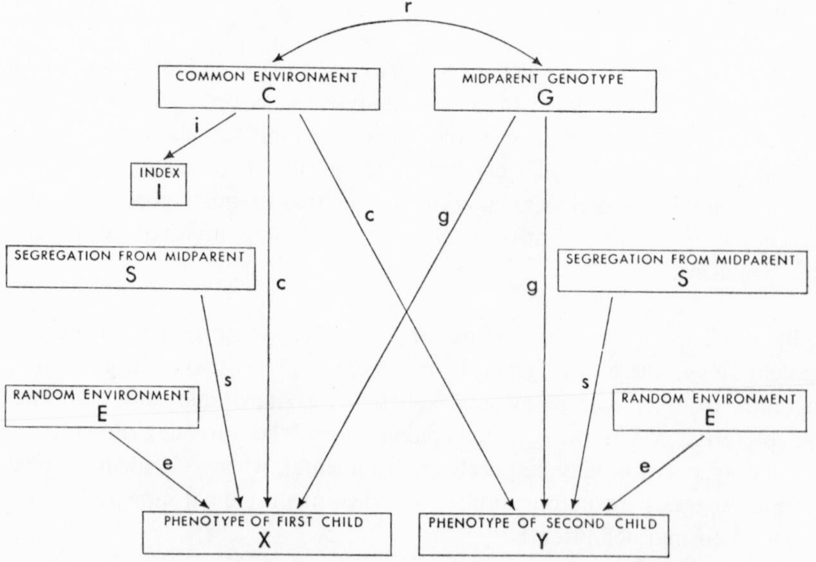

Fig. 1. Causal model of family resemblance. This simple model has been elaborated in terms of three genetic parameters and six parameters for cultural inheritance (Rao *et al.*, 1976).

for causes as well as for effects (Figure 1). The necessity for this is apparent in genetics, where the phenotype is an imperfect estimate of the genotype. Race and family environment share this imprecision. In practice the polygenic model of an indefinitely large number of additive determinants, both genetic and cultural, is assumed. The complications of dominance, epistasis, and gene-environment interaction are ignored because the system is at the limit of determinacy without them. Incomplete ascertainment and discrete variables (such as normal vs. affected) pose awkward technical difficulties. A great advantage of path analysis is that by using environmental and/or racial indices and less usual degrees of relationship (such as twins, half-sibs, and adopted children) it is feasible to resolve gene-environment covariance, biological and cultural inheritance, and genetic and environmental causes of marital correlation. Residual degrees of freedom provide a test of adequacy of the causal model. While truth may not be proven, error is given a chance to be rejected. Wright (1931) made the seminal contribution in a study of IQ. Rao *et al.* (1974, 1976) introduced indices and small-sample theory through tests of hypotheses on z transforms. The parameters change with age and may be different for maternal and paternal relationships (Rao *et al.*, 1975). They are descriptive of a particular population, with limited predictive value for altered environmental and genotypic distributions (Morton, 1974, 1975a). Nevertheless, path analysis remains the most powerful method for distinguishing between cultural and biological inheritance.

It has been usual to prefer the special case of twins over other types of relationships, including nuclear families. In part this must reflect the much simpler analysis that is possible within pairs of the same age, but the cost of such simplification is enormous. Not only are the data more difficult to collect, but information about environment common to sibs and other parameters of family resemblance is sacrificed. At every point of the analysis, the possibility that twins are in some important respect different from single births must be considered. If the object of the exercise is to make inferences about single births, then twin studies are at best a supplement to nuclear family studies.

Schull *et al.* (1970) have advocated "family sets" consisting of a randomly selected individual, a sib, a first cousin, a spouse, and a matched unrelated person. This diminishes but does not eliminate the need for covariance analysis. The difference between members of a family set for a trait of interest is regressed on a measure of kinship, providing a test of the null hypothesis that genetic relationship is unimportant, given that common environment is unimportant. With respect to parametrization of genetic and cultural inheritance and power to detect gene-environment covariance, common environment, and other complications, including a major locus, family sets are not competitive with path and segregation analysis.

Segregation analysis does not exploit the information in indices and in less usual degrees of relationship, and therefore cannot provide as rigorous a separation of biological and cultural inheritance. It is more sensitive to failure of distributional assumptions, but it is the only method able to resolve major loci, for which it provides a specific test by including terms for polygenic inheritance and environment common to sibs (MacLean *et al.*, 1975; Morton and MacLean, 1974). Assuming a null gene frequency, it gives estimates of variance components comparable to path analysis under a simplified model but accommodating incomplete ascertainment and/or qualitative data.

Segregation analysis may be supplemented by tests of distributional assumptions and linkage. Analysis of skewness and admixture in phenotypic distributions can suggest *megaphenic* effects (i.e., large relative to the standard deviation) but cannot distinguish genetic and environmental mechanisms (MacLean *et al.*, 1976). Linkage of a quantitative or qualitative trait to a Mendelian marker is often advocated for confirmation of a major locus, but this has not proven fruitful so far in man. Of course, once segregation analysis has demonstrated a major locus, it becomes reasonable to map it, but not primarily to confirm the segregation evidence which should be decisive in its own right. Unless the major locus is clear-cut, linkage evidence cannot be either convincing or useful. For example, if we knew with certainty that a major locus for intelligence were linked to the ABO system, I do not see how this information might be exploited unless segregants could be classified with little error.

Among variations of segregation analysis, the principal one opposes the greater power of large pedigrees against the simplifying assumptions which must be made if pedigree analysis is to be feasible. These include neglect of cultural inheritance, polygenes, and the mode of ascertainment. Therefore segregation analysis of pedigrees gains power, but only at the cost of accepting more spurious major loci. A reasonable compromise is to partition a large pedigree into nuclear families for the purpose of testing a major locus. Gene frequency may be enriched by a sampling of relatives, but the analysis remains valid and conservative. Then, if cultural inheritance and polygenes are found to be negligible, the pedigree may be kept intact for linkage tests, to which the mode of ascertainment is not critical and for which the power of multi-generation data is consequential. Perhaps in the future segregation analysis of pedigrees under the mixed model will become feasible.

Despite these reservations about complex segregation analysis on the null hypothesis of no polygenic or cultural inheritance, a few claims appear convincing. They include pedigrees of hyper-β-lipoproteinemia (Schrott *et al.*, 1972) and hypertriglyceridemia (Namboodiri *et al.*, 1975), where displacement due to the major locus is large. Evidence on hyperuricemia, hyperglycemia, and other quantitative traits is less clear.

Recurrence Risks

It has been customary to estimate empiric risks for complex inheritance. Herndon (1962) reminds us that *empiric* means, among other things, "one who deviates from the rules of science or accepted practice" and "one who relies upon practical experience alone, disregarding all theoretical and philosophic considerations; hence a quack, a charlatan." The danger that empiric risks acquire this derived meaning comes from increasing emphasis on client attitudes and responses, praiseworthy in itself if not diminishing concern for reliability. It is a fair reflection of the field that recent books like "Ethical issues in human genetics: genetic counseling and the use of genetic knowledge" (Hilton *et al.*, 1973) do not consider tolerances on recurrence risks either an ethical or a practical problem. While it is true that practical decisions do not depend on the third significant figure of either a recurrence risk or a laboratory result, there is a fine line between such sophistry and charlatanism. The assumption that errors are negligible gives genetic counselors a comfortable feeling, but it could only be supported by comparison with a reliable standard.

Such a standard is provided by fitting a complex model to segregation data. Within the range of common situations, the number of parameters estimated guarantees fidelity of recurrence risks, whether the underlying model is oversimplified or not. Of course, rare situations may be less accurately predicted, but for them strictly empiric risks would be based on too few cases to be trustworthy. Among the advantages of making recurrence risks an outcome of segregation analysis are that numbers of normal as well as affected relatives are considered, that a quantitative trait may be used, and that partial data on liability (such as sex and age) may be incorporated into a specific risk.

Early experience with this approach was based on simple models which included either polygenes or a major locus, but not both (Table 1). Common environment was neglected. Where determinants were poorly resolved (as was generally the case), this led to presentation of two alternate recurrence risks (Morton *et al.*, 1971). A mixed model which includes several mechanisms does not have this inconvenience (Table 2). For diseases with markedly different incidence in males and females or with any other grouping into risk categories, specific risks are provided by a liability indicator with zero mean (like ± 1 for sex) and a parameter to shift the threshold for affection.

Some genetic counselors may still prefer strictly empiric risks which pool families of different compositions (thereby creating an awkward dependence on the distribution of sibship size) and do not use quantitative traits. I know of no circumstance where this approach would be expected to give more reliable risks than those predicted from segregation analysis.

TABLE 1. The probability that an isolated case of limb-girdle muscular dystrophy be sporadic if there are s normal sibs (Morton and Chung, 1959).

S	0	4	8	—
Q	0.41	0.64	0.82	1

Diagnostic improvements since this study was carried out may have reduced the proportion of sporadic cases, an unknown fraction of which are due to heterozygous expression of usually recessive genes. The current frequency of sporadic cases is not well established.

TABLE 2. Recurrence risks for sociofamilial mental retardation (IQ<70) normal × normal matings (MacLean, 1976).

		Number of normal SIBS		
		0	2	8
Number of affected	1	0.09	0.07	0.05
SIBS	5	0.36	0.31	0.22

GENE-ENVIRONMENT INTERACTIONS

Path and segregation analysis ignore gene-environment interactions, dominance, and epistasis, yet genetics provides innumerable examples of these phenomena. Does this mean that human biometrical genetics has no firm foundation, as Lewontin (1974) has argued? The answer is to be found by considering cases where such effects do and don't appear.

Many gene-environment interactions take place in time (as when a detrimental gene becomes favorable) or space (e.g., selection against Hb^S in the absence of hyperendemic falciparum malaria). Others involve rare alleles and environments (as atypical serum cholinesterase $E^a{}_1$ and exposure to suxamethonium). Within a population at a given time, the variance due to gene-environment interaction may be negligible.

More generally, interactions enter into family resemblance in a way that is indistinguishable from the components due to random and common environment, especially the former, and so the correlation of relatives is reduced. Since the purpose of family analysis is to explain resemblance rather than dissimilarity, presence of gene-environment interaction is of no concern so long as the analysis is purely descriptive or is limited to prediction in the neighborhood of the population mean.

Dominance and epistasis (gene interaction) enter analysis of family resemblance as deviations from the best-fitting additive model, where current population parameters are used to assure a good fit. While prediction far from the population mean is hazardous, experience in biometrical genetics argues against important contributions to variance from dominance and epistasis. Recognized heterozygotes tend to be intermediate between homozygotes, as with red cell acid phosphatase where most of the genetic variance is due to a single locus. We therefore consider that omitting dominance from the analysis is less serious than failure to recognize environment common to sibs, with which dominance is usually confounded.

Recently we had an opportunity to test the assumption that interactions and dominance have negligible effects on analysis of family resemblance. Cavalli-Sforza and Feldman (1973) had simulated cultural inheritance in terms of a major locus with effects on environment of children. Their model included an arbitary degree of dominance and interaction. However, linear path analysis never appreciably overestimated heritability and did surprisingly well for environment common to sibs (Rao and Morton, 1974). We consider that interaction poses no problem for analysis of family resemblance and challenge our critics to devise a counterexample.

Inbreeding Effects

As a young student with the Atomic Bomb Casualty Commission, I examined data on effects of consanguineous marriage in Hiroshima and Nagasaki. It was clear that manifestation of rare recessives follows a Poisson process such that the probability of nonaffection is

$$S = e^{-(A+BF)}$$

where

F = inbreeding coefficient
A = panmictic load
B = inbred load.

On returning to Wisconsin I learned from Crow that Haldane (1937) had provided a theorem for relating affection to the mutation rate and from Muller that he had considered the same problem in Arner's (1908) study of consanguineous marriages. The result was a paper by Morton, Cow, and Muller (1956) on "an estimate of the mutational damage in man from data on consanguineous marriages."

Crow was most interested in separating loads due to mutation and balanced selection. His argument on the B/A ratio generated bitter controversy, largely by confusion between theory which related to total fitness and data on components of fitness. Bruce Wallace's (1970) critical book *Genetic Load* introduced consanguinity in the last few pages. A generation of biologists is now growing up who have no idea that genetic loads are inseparable from inbreeding effects. However, it was a friendly hand that inadvertently dealt the hardest blow to genetic loads. Kimura was intrigued by Haldane's (1957) cost of substitution, which under certain unlikely assumptions placed an upper limit on the rate of adaptive evolution. Kimura (1960) renamed this cost the "substitution load," and this integral over time joined the several loads which had been named but were for the most part not estimable. When it became clear that deductions from this theory were wrong (Morton, 1964), it seemed as if the superstructure of genetic loads was rotten, and only the foundation of inbreeding effects remained. Actually the funeral was premature, and genetic loads emerged to give estimates of mutation rates (Chapman *et al.*, 1964; Dewey *et al.*, 1965), numbers of alleles (Kerr, 1974), and the rate of molecular evolution (Morton, 1975b), which is so small as to be easily confused with mutation.

To illustrate these applications, consider the relation between radiosensitivity and quantity of DNA per haploid genome (Figure 2) discussed by Abrahamson *et al.* (1973). It appears that the mutation rate to markedly

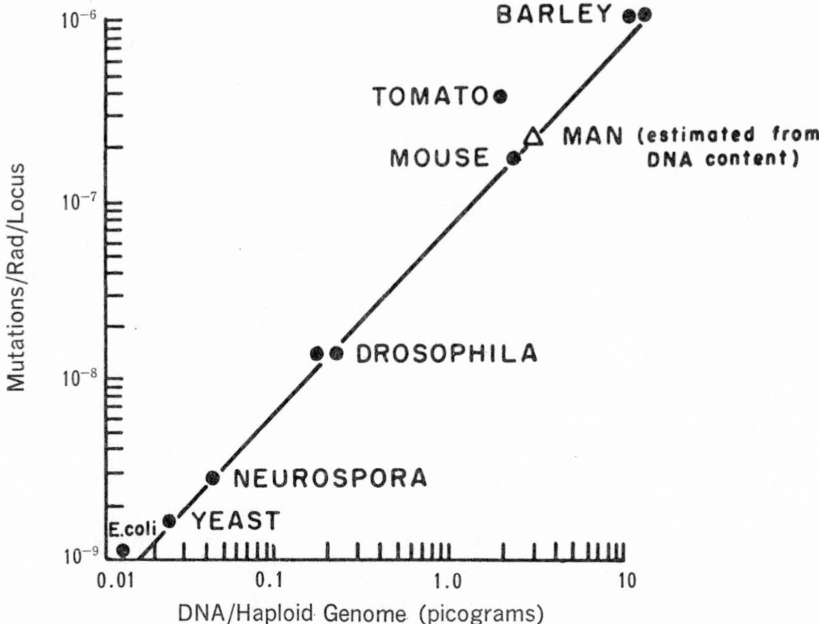

FIG. 2. Relation between forward mutation rate per locus per rad and the DNA content per haploid genome (Abrahamson *et al.*, 1973).

detrimental marker phenotypes is 2.6×10^{-7} per locus per rad. This implies that the acute doubling dose is 40 rad if the average spontaneous mutation rate is 10^{-5} per locus or 4 rad if the average rate is 10^{-6}. Smaller values are ruled out. The radiation response of the sex ratio has been estimated by genetic load theory as 1.6, 1.7, and 2.3×10^{-4} sex-linked recessive lethal mutations per gamete per r in the rat, mouse, and man (from the data of Hiroshima and Nagasaki), respectively (Havenstein *et al.*, 1968; Morton, 1960). The ratio to the per-locus rate in man is 885 lethal-producing loci per X chromosome, or 15,000 per gamete. This is part of the evidence that mammals have about 10^4 loci at which recessive lethals can occur.

Despite such applications to outbred populations, the main use of genetic load theory continues to be in analysis of inbreeding effects. Gene interactions would introduce quadratic and higher-order terms in F, but such effects have been shown to be surprisingly small (Crow, 1968). Most of the inbred load expressed as morbidity and mortality is due to genes of large effect, acting independently, and only a fraction—estimated by Crow (1968) as at most 12 percent—is caused by minor detrimentals.

The total inbred load expressed as mortality is about 1 lethal equivalent, and the additional load expressed as morbidity (but probably as mortality under primitive conditions) is about 1 detrimental equivalent (Morton, 1975b). Taking the harmonic mean of the elimination rate as .02 (Morton, Crow, and Muller, 1956), the detrimental mutation rate per gamete is .04, or perhaps two to three times that if genes affecting fertility and early embryonic mortality are included. Since Drosophila data indicate 10^4 effective loci, the mutation rate per locus/generation may be about 10^{-5} and the doubling dose is 40 r, in good agreement with other evidence. Something like 5 percent of liveborns are affected with serious monogenic disorders.

Much lower estimates are obtained from malformation registries (Trimble and Doughty, 1974), even when mild defects are included (Stevenson, 1959). Registration subsumes diagnosis, classification as monogenic, and reporting: incompleteness of any of these stages leads to underestimation of incidence. In particular, a large fraction of genetic disorders are indistinguishable by present diagnostic techniques from phenocopies and multifactorial traits.

Recently Trimble and Doughty (1974) have called attention to the much lower frequency of disease attributed to dominant genes in the British Columbia registry than in an earlier study by Stevenson (1959) which included trivial anomalies like polydactyly, hammer toe, and variations in tooth number, where dominance is questionable and registration unlikely. They concluded that estimates of "the risk to human health from these diseases, due to to an artificially induced increase in mutation rate in man, may be some 12 times too high." Such a technical point about diagnosis, classification, and reporting of some obscure anomalies is easily misunderstood. Gordon Allen (1975) hastily inferred that the new estimate reduces by one order of magnitude the expected impact of any artificial increase in human mutation rates. This, of course, is unfortunately not true, since genes with high penetrance in heterozygotes are such a small fraction of expressed genetic loads that they could be omitted or multiplied by an order of magnitude without appreciably altering expressed loads or estimates of mutation hazards.

OUTCROSSING EFFECTS

Outcrossing is a more complicated phenomenon than inbreeding. Besides increased heterozygosity and therefore lower morbidity from recessive genes, outcrosses (especially after the first generation) have the potential to form new genetic combinations not previously exposed to the sieve of natural selection. To consider a simple case, the Kell allele is polymorphic in Caucasians, and the Sutter allele is polymorphic in Negroes. Only mulattos have appreciable frequencies of K/k^s heterozygotes. Such novel genotypes, apart from their utility to the biologist, have some epidemiological interest. For example, cystic fibrosis is a recessive gene polymorphic in Caucasians and is rare in other populations. Because of heterozygosity, outcrosses have low affection rates (Figure 3), as expected (Wright and Morton, 1968).

Outcrossing studies for more complex diseases require a huge sample

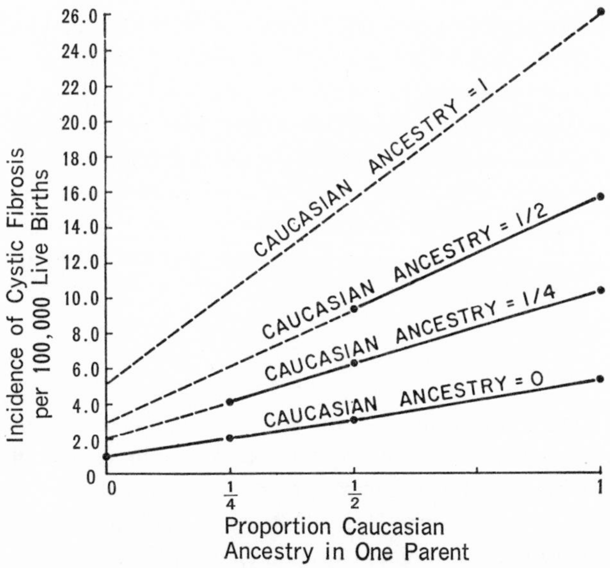

FIG. 3. Incidence of cystic fibrosis per 100,000 live births in unmixed and hybrid matings. On the abscissa, the proportion of Caucasian ancestry may vary from 0 to 1 for one of the parents. For the other parent, the proportion of Caucasian ancestry is fixed at 1 value. Calculated on the assumption of a single locus (Wright and Morton, 1968).

from a population in which the ethnic groups and their hybrids cohabit in as homogeneous an environment as possible. Brazil and Hawaii approximate this condition. For mortality, morbidity, and size there is no significant outcrossing effect attributable to heterozygosity or recombination (Morton *et al.*, 1967). Expressing biological effects as an equivalent inbreeding coefficient, this is $.0005 \pm .0015$ for minor ethnic differences (like Japanese and Korean) and $.0009 \pm .0014$ for major differences (like Caucasian and Oriental). These estimates are much smaller than for polymorphic genes, which give .18 as the kinship of major races (Morton and Van Wierst, 1976). Some simulation studies give even higher values, which, however, are based on arbitrary assumptions.

Bresler (1970) has reported a recombination effect on fetal death in a small anamnestic sample. Since no suggestion of this was found in the much larger Hawaiian study, it is likely that some artifact, such as a correlation between completeness of genealogies and abortion histories, explains Bresler's results (Freire-Maia *et al.*, 1974).

At the level of isolate-breaking, outcrossing effects are best studied in terms of Malécot's (1948) concept of isolation by distance. Morton *et al.* (1973) showed effects for rare genes in Switzerland. Metrical traits have given conflicting results, presumably reflecting small levels of kinship, on the one hand, and environmental heterogeneity on the other. Furusho (1965) noted that decrease of height with marital distance in Japan is an artifact of lower stature in the northern and southern extremes of the country. Such problems must be borne in mind when assessing reports of heterosis due to isolate-breaking in man (Hulse, 1957; Wolanski *et al.*, 1970).

Group Differences

The same populations which permit studies of outcrossing allow group comparisons. Control of environmental variables is more difficult than for outcrossing, where additive parental effects can be used as covariates. Path analysis offers some promise (Li, 1975) especially when combined with racial and environmental indices (Morton *et al.*, 1976).

This approach is illustrated by data on academic performance in Hawaii (Figure 4). Unlike the mainland data of the Coleman report, these data show that race is not a significant determinant of performance. Hawaii is the only American state in which schools are not governed by local boards,

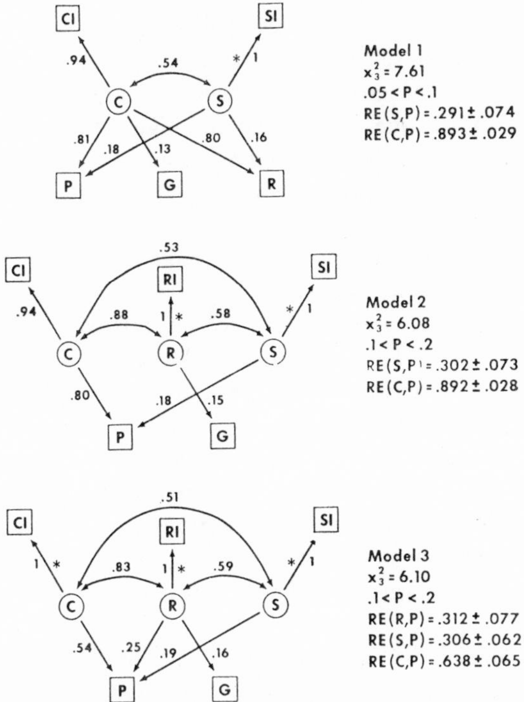

FIG. 4. Causal models of academic performance in Hawaii. P=performance, G=grade (a measure of increase in performance with age), R=race, S=social class, S=school, I=index. Note that racial characteristics are consistent with determination by class and school, and do not have a significant effect on performance. Only social class has a large effect and relative direct effect (RE) on performance (Morton, Stout, and Fisher, 1976).

which perpetuate class and ethnic norms. Even in Hawaii, only 30 percent of the effect of school characteristics on academic performance is exerted directly, the remainder being due to covariance between institutional characteristics and social class of the attendance area. Conversely, almost 90 percent of the large class effect on performance is exerted directly. The difficulty of testing genetic hypotheses against the overpowering noise of family environment is obvious, especially on the American mainland. Critical genetic evidence could only come from family resemblance in a hybrid population. The voice of unreason is strong enough to suppress such studies on cognition in the foreseeable future.

The intemperance of self-styled liberals has so far been less effective in preventing studies of group differences for noncognitive traits. It is still permissible to ask questions about the high rate of cystic fibrosis in Caucasians, harelip in Orientals, talipes equinovarus in Polynesians, or hypertension in North American Blacks. We understand the genetic mechanism for cystic fibrosis, although there is no consensus about how that recessive gene reached polymorphic frequency in northwest Europe. The genetic basis of ethnic differences for harelip and talipes equinovarus seems demonstrated by their persistence in related populations under different environments. The heavy impact of hypertension on North American Blacks remains mysterious. Diet, stress, and genes have their advocates. Krieger (1970) found no evidence of a racial difference in a hybrid Brazilian population, to which we are now applying recent advances in path analysis in the hope of resolving biological and environmental determinants of blood pressure. Infant mortality due to congenital malformation is a clear precedent for nongenetic group differences (Figure 5). In this field, as in all others, genetic explanations should wait for genetic evidence.

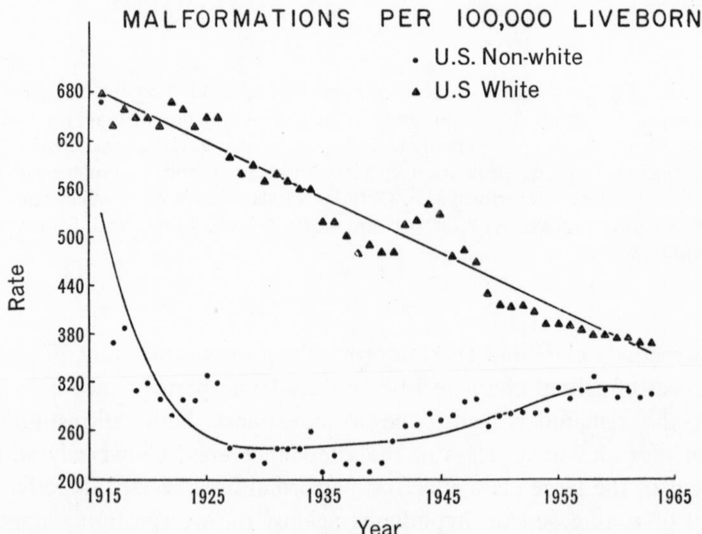

Fig. 5. Infant deaths ascribed to congenital malformations per 100,000 liveborns (Morton *et al.*, 1976).

Population Surveillance

Human populations are increasingly exposed to novel agents which may be mutagens, teratogens, or carcinogens. Programs of surveillance for these hazards have characteristically stressed ingenious manipulations of bacteria, which may or may not be relevant to man. Those who have addressed the human condition usually assume a prospective cytological study. For diseases with a high ascertainment probability, the efficiency of a surveillance program may be increased a thousand-fold by sequential analysis in an appropriate registry. Here efficiency is measured by the number of individuals who must be examined to detect a given hazard. If the disease has an incidence of $1/x$, then a registry of affected individuals is x times as efficient as a prospective study. Sequential analysis typically requires only half as many observations as a fixed-sample size test with the same Type I and II errors. Therefore the efficiency of this type of surveillance is roughly $2x$ as great as a prospective study with fixed sample size, or at least 1000-fold for Down's syndrome. We have demonstrated the feasibility of population surveillance for such conditions (Morton and Lindsten, 1976). Table 3 shows a sequential test on Down's syndrome in Sweden. During a six-year period it terminated twice with the reassuring decision "no increase." Setting the Type I and II error at .1, the test on a population of this size would be expected to detect a 12 percent increase in frequency.

I believe that this method of sequential population surveillance should be incorporated into every serious program to detect mutagenic, teratogenic, and carcinogenic hazards. The advantages of sequential surveillance are not limited to the fact that it requires much smaller expected sample sizes for given Type I and II errors. In addition, it provides a surveillance pro-

TABLE 3. A sequential test on Down's syndrome in Sweden ($\alpha=\beta=.1$, $K=1.116$).

Year	Observed	Expected	Lod_e	Decision
1968	165	144.3	1.37	Continue
1969	131	137.4	− .19	"
1970	142	140.6	− .92	"
1971	135	144.9	−2.91	Accept H_0
1972	137	142.0	−1.44	Continue
1973	138	138.8	−2.39	Accept H_0

tocol, with sufficiently frequent decisions (to continue sampling, make supplementary tests, and accept or reject the null hypothesis) that a registry becomes more than a shoebox full of unanalyzed data. Sequential tests can contribute to the quality of a registry, to the morale of its investigations, and to the value of a surveillance program to the population being monitored.

Dynamics of Genes Predisposing to Common Disease

Genetic epidemiology overlaps population genetics, but it does not include theoretical studies directed toward evolutionary biology. It is, however, broad enough to consider the causes of unusual concentrations of genes predisposing to disease.

For common diseases such concentrations seem paradoxical, since natural selection might be expected to reduce their frequency. In such cases it is tempting to speculate that stable polymorphism is maintained by other selective forces or that the polymorphism is transient. Genetic drift to high frequency is difficult to prove or disprove in populations now large, but small many generations ago. Alternatively, appeal may be made to the "thrifty genotype" hypothesis of Neel (1962). As originally proposed for diabetes, this hypothesis states that a transient polymorphism with advantage for an uncommon allele in homozygotes shifts to diasdvantage in an altered environment. However, homozygous advantage in any environment for what are now pathological levels of hyperglycemia and hypercholesterolemia seems to me unlikely, and so I prefer a different formulation which Neel (1962, p. 359) also advanced but did not favor. Suppose that under more primitive conditions a gene G conferred an advantage in heterozygotes, with relative fitness $1-s$, 1, and $1-t$ in the genotypes GG, GG′, and G′G′, respectively ($0<s$, $t<1$). The effect of the locus on population fitness is the "segregation load" $st/(s+t)$, which is about .1 for sickle cell disease under hyperendemic malaria. I have argued elsewhere that the segregation load for the average locus is less than 10^{-4} (Morton, 1975b). This implies weak selection which may be "plastic" in different environments (Morton *et al.*, 1966). If the environment changes so that the gene is unfavorable even in heterozygotes, we have an illustration of gene-environment interaction and the paradox of a common disease caused by a genetic polymorphism once thrifty but now pathogenic. Alternatively, a gene causing disease in middle or old age may be favorable at an earlier stage of the life cycle. A gene never advantageous, but held in the population by a balance of mutation against weak selection, may become more detrimental in a changed environment. With any of these models, commonness is no insuperable objection to a major gene hypothesis. Therefore a polygenic model should be preferred only if supported by segregation analysis, and not because of any argument on evolutionary grounds against a major gene predisposing to common disease.

Relaxation of selection (for example by improved medical care) has effects which depend critically on the unknown factors which have maintained genes predisposing to disease. If there is opposition between mutation and selection, the gene frequencies will increase for a long time to reach a new equilibrium. If there is balance between selection forces, some of which are independent of the disease, then the gene frequency will increase for only a few generations. We can deduce the consequences of different models, but to determine the dynamics in a particular case is much more difficult and will require more than one generation.

Summary

The development of genetic epidemiology has been reviewed, and the following aspects have been discussed: familial resemblance, recurrence risks, gene-environment interactions, inbreeding and outcrossing effects, group comparisons, population surveillance, and dynamics of genes predisposing to common disease. Although genetic epidemiology is barely 20 years old, it has matured into an exciting discipline which promises to enrich both epidemiology and genetics.

REFERENCES

Abrahamson, S., Bender, M. A., Conger, A. D., and Wolff, S. 1973. The uniformity of radiation-induced mutation rates among different species. *Nature* **245**: 460–462.

Allen, G. 1975. Periodical abstracts. *Soc. Biol.* **22**: 199

Arner, G. B. L. 1908. Consanguineous marriages in the American population. *Columbia Univ. Studies Hist. Econ. Public Law* **31(3)**: 1–99.

Blumberg, B. S. 1961. *Genetic polymorphisms and geographic variation in disease.* Grune & Stratton, New York, U.S.A.

Bresler, J. 1970. Outcrossings in Caucasians and fetal loss. *Soc. Biol.* **17**: 17–25.

Cavalli-Sforza, L. L., and Feldman, M. W. 1973. Cultural versus biological inheritance: Phenotypic transmission from parents to children (a theory of the effect of parental phenotypes on children's phenotypes). *Am. J. Hum. Genet.* **25**: 618–637.

Chapman, A. B., Hansen, J. L., Haverstein, G. B., and Morton, N. E. 1964. Genetic effects of cumulative irradiation on prenatal and early postnatal survival in the rat. *Genetics* **50**: 1029–1042.

Crow, J. F. 1968. Some analyses of hidden variability in Drosophila populations. *In* Lewontin, R. C. (Ed.), *Population biology and evolution.* University Press, Syracuse, N.Y., U.S.A., pp. 71–86.

Dewey, W. J., Barrai, I., Morton, N. E., and Mi, M. P. 1965. Recessive genes in severe mental defect. *Am. J. Hum. Genet.* **17**: 237–256.

Freire-Maia, A., Stevenson, C., and Morton, N. E. 1974. Hybridity effect on mortality. *Soc. Biol.* **21**: 232–234.

Furusho, T. 1965. Relationship of the stature of the child to the distance between parental birthplaces. *Jap. J. Hum. Genet.* **10**: 22–38.

Haldane, J. B. S. 1937. The effect of variation on fitness. *Amer. Naturalist.* **71**: 337–349.

Haldane, J. B. S. 1957. The cost of natural selection. *J. Genet.* **55**: 511–524.

Havenstein, G. B., Taylor, B. A., Hansen, J. C., Morton, N. E., and Chapman, A. B. 1968. Genetic effects of cumulative X-irradiation on the secondary sex ratio of the laboratory rat. *Genetics* **59**: 255–274.

Herndon, C. N. 1962. Empiric risks. *In* Burdette, G. (Ed.), *Methodology in human genetics.* Holden-Day, San Francisco, U.S.A., pp. 144–155.

Hilton, B., Callahan, D., Harris, M., Condliffe, P., and Berkley, B. 1973. *Ethical issues in human genetics. Genetic counseling and the use of genetic knowledge.* Plenum, New York, U.S.A.

Hulse, F. S. 1957. Exogamie et heterosis. *Arch. Suisses Anthrop. Gener.* **22**: 103–125.

Kerr, W. E. 1974. Advances in cytology and genetics of bees. *Ann. Rev. Ent.* **19**: 253–268.

Kimura, M. 1960. Optimum mutation rate and degree of dominance as determined by the principle of minimum genetic load. *J. Genet.* **57**: 21–34.

Krieger, H. 1970. Racial admixture effects in northeastern Brazil. *Ann. Hum. Genet.* **33**: 423–428.

Lewontin, R. C. 1974. Annotation: The analysis of variance and the analysis of causes. *Am. J. Hum. Genet.* **26**: 400–411.

Li, C. C. 1975. *Path analysis—a primer.* Boxwood Press, Pacific Grove, Calif., U.S.A.

MacLean, C. J. 1976. Recurrence risks for mental retardation (in preparation)

MacLean, C. J., Morton, N. E., and Lew, R. 1975. Analysis of family resemblance. IV. Operational characteristics of segregation analysis. *Am. J. Hum. Genet.* **27**: 365–384.

MacLean, C. J., Morton, N. E., Elston, R. C., and Yee, S. 1976. Skewness in commingled distributions. *Biometrics* **32**: 695–699.

Malécot, G. 1948. *Les mathématiques de l'hérédite*. Masson, Paris, France.

Morton, N. E. 1960. The mutational load due to detrimental genes in man. *Am. J. Hum. Genet.* **12**: 348–364.

Morton, N. E. 1964. Models and evidence in human population genetics. *In* Geerts, S. J. (Ed.), *Genetics today*. Proc. XI Intern. Congr. Gen., The Hague, Netherlands; Pergamon Press, Oxford, England, pp. 936–951.

Morton, N. E. 1974. Analysis of family resemblance. I. Introduction. *Am. J. Hum. Genet.* **26**: 318–330.

Morton, N. E. 1975a. Analysis of family resemblance and group differences. *Soc. Biol.* **22**: 111–116.

Morton, N. E. 1975b. Kinship, fitness and evolution. *In* Salzano, F. M. (Ed.) *The role of natural selection in human evolution.* North Holland, Amsterdam, pp. 133–154.

Morton, N. E., and Chung, C. S. 1959. Formal genetics of muscular dystrophy. *Am. J. Hum. Genet.* **11**: 360–379.

Morton, N. E., and Lindsten, J. 1976. Surveillance of Down's syndrome as a paradigm of population monitoring. *Hum. Hered.* (in press).

Morton, N. E., and MacLean, C. J. 1974. Analysis of family resemblance. III. Complex segregation of quantitative traits. *Am. J. Hum. Genet.* **26**: 489–503.

Morton, N. E., and Van Wierst B. 1976. Human microdifferentiation in the Western Pacific.

Morton, N. E., Chung, C. S., and Mi, M. P. 1967. *Genetics of interracial crosses in Hawaii.* Karger, Basel, Switzerland.

Morton, N. E., Crow, J. F., and Muller H. J. 1956. An estimate of the mutational damage in man from data on consanguineous marriage. *Proc. Natl. Acad. Sci.* **42**: 855–863.

Morton, N. E., Krieger, H., and Mi, M. P. 1966. Natural selection on polymorphism in northeastern Brasil. *Am. J. Hum. Genet.* **18**: 153–171.

Morton, N. E., Stout, W. T., and Fischer, C. 1976. Academic performance in Hawaii. *Soc. Biol.* **23**: 13–20.

Morton, N. E., Yee, S., and Lew R. 1971. Complex segregation analysis. *Am. J. Hum Genet.* **23**: 602–611.

Morton, N. E., Klein, D., Hussels, I. E., Dodinval, P., Todorov, A., Lew, R., and Yee, S. 1973. Genetic structure of Switzerland. *Am. J. Hum. Genet.* **25**: 347–361.

Namboodiri, K. K., Elston, R. C., Glueck, C. J., Fallat, R., Bucher, C. R., and Tsang, R. 1975. Bivariate analyses of cholesterol and triglyceride levels in families in which probands have type IIb lipoprotein phenotype. *Am. J. Hum. Genet.* **27**: 454–471.

Neel, J. V. 1962. Diabetes mellitus: A "thrifty" genotype rendered detrimental by "progress"? *Am. J. Hum. Genet.* **14**: 353–362.

Neel, J. V. and Schull, W. J. 1954. *Hum. Hered.* U. Chicago Press, Chicago, U.S.A.

Neel, J. V., Shaw, M. W., and Schull, W. J. 1965. *Genetics and the epidemiology of chronic diseases*. U.S.D.H.E.W., Public Health Service Publ. 1163.

Rao, D. C., and Morton, N. E. 1974. Path analysis of family resemblance in the presence of gene environment interaction. *Am. J. Hum. Genet.* **26**: 767–772.

Rao, D. C., Morton, N. E., and Yee, S. 1974. Analysis of family resemblance. II. A linear model for familial correlation. *Am. J. Hum. Genet.* **26**: 331–359.

Rao, D. C., Morton, N. E., and Yee, S. 1976. Resolution of cultural and biological inheritance by path analysis. *Am. J. Hum. Genet.* **28**: 228–242.

Rao, D. C., MacLean, C. J., Morton, N. E., and Yee, S. 1975. Analysis of family resemblance. V. Height and weight in northeastern Brazil. *Am. J. Hum. Genet.* **27**: 509–520.

Schrott, H. G., Goldstein, J. L., Hazzard, W. R., McGoodwin, M. M., and Motulsky, A. G. 1972. Familial hypercholesterolemia in a large kindred. Evidence for a monogenic mechanism. *Ann. Int. Med.* **76**: 711–720.

Schull, W. J., Harburg, E., Erfurt, J. C., Schork, M. A., and Rice, R. 1970. A family set method for estimating heredity and stress. II. Preliminary results of the genetic methodology in a pilot survey of negro blood pressure, Detroit, 1966–1967. *J. Chron. Dis.* **23**: 83–92.

Stevenson, A. C. 1959. The load of hereditary defects in human populations. *Radiat. Res.*, Suppl. **1**: 306–325.

Trimble, B. K., and Doughty, J. H. 1974. The amount of hereditary disease in human populations. *Ann. Hum. Genet.* (London) **38**: 199–223.

Wallace, B. 1970. *Genetic load, its biological and conceptual aspects*. Prentice-Hall, New York, U.S.A.

Wolanski, N. E., Jarosz, E., and Pyzuk, M. 1970. Heterosis in man: Growth of offspring and distance between parents' birthplaces. *Soc. Biol.* **17**: 1–16.

Wright, S. 1931. Statistical methods in biology. *J. Am. Stat. Assoc.* **26**: 155–163.

Wright, S. W., and Morton, N. E. 1968. Genetic studies of cystic fibrosis in Hawaii. *Am. J. Hum. Genet.* **20**: 157–169.

Human Genetic Load

Takeo Maruyama

A gene with a deleterious effect is certainly a burden or "load" to an individual who carries it. The effect can be death, illness, physical weakness, sterility, and so on. The harm caused by deleterious genes can also be regarded as a burden or load to a society, for the average fitness or welfare of the society as a whole is impaired by the presence of such genes. If a society has many individuals who require medical care, it needs more doctors, hospitals, and medicines, each of which is a load which must be borne by the society; and if the cause is genetic, the result can be regarded as a genetic load.

There are numerous known hereditary traits which are caused by single or multiple mutant genes (see McKusick, 1975). Nearly all of them are to some extent harmful. Extensive experiments using fruit flies and other organisms have shown that hardly any mutant can be beneficial to a carrier, in comparison with the gene from which the mutant is derived; probably almost every newly arising mutant is inferior to its original gene. This seems to be true irrespective of the environment in which the genes are placed. Therefore a certain fraction (probably a large one) of mutant genes is harmful in any environment.

The word "load" was first used by H. J. Muller (1950) in assessing the impact of mutation on the human population. In Muller's thinking, the load was a burden, measured in terms of reduced fitness but felt in terms of death, sterility, illness, and physical and mental disability.

At present, however, in most evolutionary and population genetic considerations the concept of genetic load is used in a broader sense: It is a measure of the amount of natural selection associated with a certain amount of genetic variability. It is, then, not necessarily a burden. Consider a

National Institute of Genetics, Mishima, Japan.

situation in which the environment has changed and the normal wild type becomes inferior to a mutant. The mutant which becomes superior to the former wild type will increase in frequency and eventually spread over the whole population, but the process will require the sacrifice of the genes which are replaced. This sacrifice in the process of gene substitution is not bad for the population; it is necessary in order for a species to survive or to further evolve. Another frequently noted example is the situation where heterozygous individuals are superior to homozygotes. This creates variability and a genetic load, but the polymorphic population has a higher average fitness than it would if it were monomorphic.

Genetic Load

A mathematical definition of genetic load (Crow, 1958) is as follows: the proportion by which the fitness of the average genotype in the population is reduced in comparison with the best genotype—that is,

$$L=\frac{w_{\max}-w}{w_{\max}}$$

where w is the average fitness of the population and $w_{\max}$ is the fitness of the most fit genotype among those being considered. Thus a genetic load is defined as the amount by which the population's average fitness is impaired, or by which the incidence of specific types of morbidity, mortality, or infertility is increased, by the fact that the population is not of the optimum genotype composition. If the trait in question is survival, the genetic load can be expressed in terms of its lethal equivalent. A lethal equivalent is defined as a group of genes that, if dispersed in different individuals, causes on the average one death (e.g., one lethal gene, or two genes, each with 50 percent probability of causing death). The total load per gamete can be measured in terms of the average number of lethal equivalents in the zygote that would result from doubling the chromosomes of this gamete. Corresponding to lethal equivalents, it is also possible to measure the sterility load in terms of sterile equivalents. In man, where specific detrimental traits can be studied, the genetic load due to specific types of defects can be measured (Morton, 1960).

The genetic load can be assigned to different causes. For this purpose we define the genetic load attributable to a certain factor as the proportion by which the population fitness is decreased in comparison to what it would be if this factor were absent. Almost any factor that influences gene frequencies can lead to a change in the average fitness and therefore create a genetic load, in the sense defined by Crow. Only a few have been investigated in detail, and a convenient classification of the more important of these follows:

1. *Mutational load.* This is the amount by which the average fitness of a population is diminished by recurrent mutation. (See Haldane, 1937; Kimura, 1961.)

2. *Segregational load* (or balanced load). As mentioned above, a segregational load occurs when the fittest genotype is heterozygous. If this is the case, the heterozygous individuals will produce homozygous individuals less fit than the heterozygotes as a consequence of Mendelian segregation, and the segregational load is the decrease in fitness compared to the most fit heterozygote which would prevail if the segregation were absent. (See Dobzhansky 1955, 1957.)

3. *Substitutional load.* It is likely over time that changes in the environment may alter the relative fitnesses of genotypes so that the genotype favored prior to the change is not favored after it, and therefore that the newly favored genotype which is rare will increase and replace the previously common genotype. The load imposed upon the gene substitution has been termed the cost of natural selection or the substitutional load. (See Haldane, 1957; Kimura, 1960, 1960a; Crow, 1968). Haldane showed that the total cost (load) over the whole process of a gene substitution is determined almost entirely by the initial frequency of the mutant and hardly at all by the selective advantage of the mutant. (See also Felsenstein, 1971).

4. *Recombinational load.* If we consider two or more loci simultaneously, if the recombination results in a decrease in average fitness in comparison with a hypothetical situation where recombination is absent, we can define a recombinational load in analogy with the segregational load.

5. *Incompatibility load.* Certain genotypes may have reduced fitness with certain maternal genotypes—for example, the Rh-positive child of the Rh-negative mother. The average fitness reduction associated with this cause has been termed the incompatibility load. (See Crow and Morton, 1960.)

6. *Finite population.* In a finite population, the gene frequencies drift away from the equilibrium values expected in an infinite population. The drift away from the equilibrium usually reduces the fitness, thereby creating a genetic load. The case of frequency-dependent fitness, where the fitness of a genotype depends on its frequency in the population, was studied by

Kimura and Ohta (1970). (See also Kimura *et al.*, 1963, and Kimura and Maruyama, 1968.)

7. *Migrational load.* The fitness of a population is likely to be lowered by immigrants evolved elsewhere under other environmental conditions, thereby creating a genetic load.

There are still other types of loads which can be identified, but these appear to be those important to man. Hereafter, however, I will confine my discussion mainly to the mutational load, which seems to be of greatest importance to man.

Mutation Load

Haldane (1937) showed that the effect of mutation on population fitness depends mainly on the mutation rate and not on the harmfulness of the individual mutants. The decrease in average fitness as a consequence of recurrent mutation is equal to the total mutation rate multiplied by a factor between 1 and 2, depending on the degree of dominance. Haldane argues as follows:

> It is at once clear that in equilibrium such abnormal genes are wiped out by natural selection at exactly the same rate as they are produced by mutation. It does not matter whether the gene is lethal or almost harmless. In the first case, every individual carrying it, or if it is recessive, every individual homozygous for it, is wiped out. In the second the viability or fertility of such individuals may only be reduced by one-thousandth. In either case, however, the loss of fitness to the species depends entirely on the mutation rate and not at all on the effect of the gene upon the fitness of the individual carrying it, provided this is large enough to keep the gene rare.

Muller argued alternatively that a less harmful gene would have less chance of being eliminated by selection from the population in each generation, and therefore more individuals would be affected, while a more harmful gene has an opposite feature. Hence total genetic damage summed over all the affected individuals is independent of the harmfulness: every mutant eventually causes one genetic death. This is called the Haldane-Mueller principle.

This principle enables us to make an assessment of the amount of the mutation load in terms of the mutation rate. Here the quantity is the sum of the rates over all loci. If the question is the viability, the quantity which determines the load is the total mutation rate of loci affecting viability. In fact, it is difficult to measure the genetic load expressed in a random mating equilibrium population, and it can only be assessed through indirect means. On the other hand, it is possible to measure the genetic load which would be expressed if a population were made completely homozygous, the so-called homozygous (or inbred) load. The following argument and calculation made by Muller (1948, 1956) illustrates well the underlying principle in measuring the inbred load from data on inbred and non-inbred individual mortality. From survival data of children from first-cousin marriages and from marriages between non-relatives published by Arner (1908), Muller observed that the children from first-cousin marriages showed 83.2 percent survival up to 20 years of age, and the children from non-relative marriages showed 88.4 percent survival up to the same age. The difference is highly significant and is possibly due to genetic effect of consanguineous marriage. Dividing the former figure by the latter, we see that only 94.1 percent of those who should have survived if the parents were unrelated were able to survive if their parents were first-cousins. That is, the inbreeding resulted in the death, before 20 years of age, of about 6 percent of those who would otherwise have lived. Since first-cousin inbreeding gives only 1/16 probability of homozygosis of genes that would otherwise have been heterozygous, we may multiply this 6 percent mortality by 16. This gives 96 percent as the sum of the excess risks of genetic death that would on the average be run between birth and 20 years by hypothetical individuals who were homozygous for all the genes contained in just one of the gametes that produced them. This calculation led Muller to conclude that every person on the average contains heterozygously at least one lethal equivalent which would kill him or her between birth and maturity if it were homozygous. A similar conclusion had been stated by Arner (1908) (see also Cavalli-Sforza and Bodmer, 1971, p. 365). The above argument and calculation can be summarized as follows:

	Non-related marriages ($f=0$)	First-cousin marriages ($f=1/16$)
Actual survival rate	88.4%	83.2%
Normalized	100	94.1

$100-94.1=5.9\%$ (mortality due to inbreeding of $f=1/16$: $5.9\div(1/16)=95\%$ (expected mortality with $f=1$). Hence about one lethal equivalent/gamete.

There are numerous early efforts to use human data for estimating the average number of deleterious genes possessed by the average individual: Russel, 1952; Reed, 1954; Slatis, 1954; Penrose, 1957. But these studies did not make an attempt to inquire about how these genes were maintained in the population. In 1956, Morton, Crow, and Muller advanced a method with considerably broader objectives; this is now well known as the Morton-Crow-Muller method and is widely used. The Morton-Crow-Muller method was intended to evaluate (in addition to the homozygous load in terms of lethal equivalents) the nature of the load with respect to whether its major part is maintained by reccurrent deleterious mutations or by a balance of heterozygote superiority over homozygotes. That is, the aim of the method is to determine whether the inbred load in the population is due mainly to deleterious genes maintained by mutation pressure (the mutation load) or to genes maintained by overdominance (the segregational or overdominance load). Although I do not intend to discuss any details of the Morton-Crow-Muller method, it is necessary to review the essence of the method. If we denote by L_I the genetic load expressed when a whole population is made completely homozygous without the pressure of natural selection, and by L_R the genetic load expressed in a random mating population, Morton, Crow, and Muller have shown that

$$-\log_e S = (L_R + E) + (L_I - L_R)f$$

where S is the survival probability if the load is to be measured in terms of lethal equivalent, E is death due to environmental factors, and f is the inbreeding coefficient. (If the load is to be measured by a different quantity, the meaning of these symbols ought to be changed accordingly.) We can rewrite this equation as

$$-\log_e S = A + Bf$$

where

$$A = L_R + E$$
$$B = L_I - L_R.$$

Here the observables are the survival probability S and the inbreeding coefficient f, and the unknowns are A and B. Since the equation involves two unknowns, the solution requires data on the survival rate, S, for at least two different degrees of inbreeding. Usually $f=0$ in children of unrelated marriages and $f>0$ in children of consanguineous marriages. For children of first-cousin marriages, $f=1/16$. If we have data on the survival rate S for various values of f, we can solve the equation for A and B. Using the definitions of A and B, the quantity of our interest L_I is given by inequality

$$B = L_I - L_R \leqq L_I \leqq A + B = L_I + E.$$

Therefore the inbred load (L_I) lies between the components B and $A+B$.

Let us further examine the nature of the genetic load in relation to the estimable quantities A and B. It can be shown that for the following model of two alleles at a locus,

Genotype		AA	Aa	aa
Freq.	$f=0$	p^2	$2pq$	q^2
	$f=1$	p	0	q
Fitness	mutation selection	1	$1-sh$	$1-s$
	overdominance	$1-s_1$	1	$1-s_2$

Nature of load	Load		Ratio
	$L_R(f=0)$	$L_I(f=1)$	L_R/L_I
Mutation-selection	$\sim 2\,qsh$	sq	$1/2h$
Overdominance	$\frac{s_1 s_2}{s_1+s_2}$	$\frac{2s_1 s_2}{s_1+s_2}$	2

(See, for example, Cavalli-Sforza and Bodmer, 1971, pp. 354–358.)

Therefore the ratio of the inbred load to the random load would be $1/2h$ if the load were mainly due to deleterious mutants, and the ratio would be 2 if the load were mainly due to overdominance.

Nothing is known about the average value of the quantity h in man. There are, however, statistical and experimental estimates for lethals in *Drosophila melanogaster*, giving $h=0.02$ to 0.03 (Hiraizumi and Crow, 1960; Crow and Temin, 1964). The extrapolation from *Drosophila* to man can clearly be questioned. However, if we accept this as an average estimate of h, the ratio of the inbred load to the random load would be on the average on the order of $15\sim25$, and therefore quite large. On the other hand, the ratio of the inbred load to the random load in the overdominance case would be 2 and thus much lower than the ratio in the former case. Here we assumed two alleles maintained by overdominance in which the ratio L_I/L_R is 2, but in general if there were k mutually overdominant alleles, the ratio would be k, which can be larger than 2. Therefore the L_I/L_R ratio is not necessarily 2, but it is also unlikely to be very large, because the possibility of having a large number of mutually overdominant alleles at every locus must be small. Hence in theory it is expected that if the load is maintained by mutation and selection balance, the ratio will be large, whereas if the load is due to overdominance, the ratio will be small. Of course, in practice, reliable data will be required to estimate the ratio accurately. Morton (1961) has observed high (B/A) ratios for a number of phenotypes whose frequencies and genetic behavior indicate that they are mostly due to recessive genes maintained primarily by mutation pressure: low-grade mental deficiency, 46.1; recessive muscular dystrophy, 225.9; recessive deaf-mutism, 442.0. However, even if the inbred load is maintained by mutation-selection pressure, the L_I/L_R ratio need not be necessarily high, since h may be large. In fact, as I will discuss later, in *Drosophila* a large class of deleterious genes with slight effect is known to have a high average value for (and so a high) B/A ratio h, yet this class of mutants is believed to be maintained by mutation pressure (Mukai *et al.*, 1974).

Thus the Morton-Crow-Muller method is an important tool in estimating the inbred genetic load and also in determining whether the major part of the inbred load is due to the mutation selection balance or to the overdominance balance. At first Morton, Crow, and Muller applied their method to human data from France and the United States, and concluded that the load expressed in inbred individuals is mainly mutational. But as far as I know, subsequent studies, from both the theoretical viewpoint and the results of data analysis, indicate that a conclusion about whether the inbred load is mainly mutational or segregational has not been reached.

Schull and Neel (1965) conducted one of the most thorough analyses presently available on the homozygous load in man. They used data from diverse sources and diverse in nature; and the load expressed in terms of lethal equivalents from their findings is summarized in Table 1. The following passage from Schull and Neel (1965, pp. 346–348) gives a good account of the present situation regarding the human mutational load:

> Perusal of this table reveals certain obvious inconsistencies—negative B/A ratios, to cite one. But there is an over-all element of agreement which, in respect of the aforementioned dissimilarities in the studies and the marked differences in medical practice, nutrition, and so on in the areas for which the data are reported, might be viewed as unexpected. Thus, for example, we note that with one exception, namely, the

TABLE 1.* Summary of lethal equivalents as estimated for various stages of manifestation in contemporary populations. The column headed "Total" represents the sum of lethal equivalents manifesting themselves as stillbirths or deaths between parturition and maturity.

Country and/or population	Lethal equivalents: Miscarriage	Stillbirth	Neonatal death	Infantile and juvenile death	Total	B/A
Brazil:						
Indians				1.37[a]	1.37	0.71
Negroes	3.20	1.24		1.38[a]	2.62	9.22
Whites	−0.59	0.88		−0.20[a]	0.68	0.18
France:						
Finistère		0.38	0.68	2.44	3.50	
Loir-et-Cher		0.29	0.48	1.93	2.70	18.53
Morbihan		1.07	1.15	2.18	4.40	
Germany					0.86[b]	1.77
Italy			1.03[c]	2.06	3.09	8.37
Japan:						
Fukushima					0.96[b]	5.85
Hiroshima		0.14	0.29	0.63	1.06	6.08
Hoshino		0.15	0.67		0.82	10.57
Mishima		0.26	−0.29	0.55	0.52	1.58
Nagasaki		−0.02	0.20	0.15	0.33	1.08
Shizuoka					1.11[b]	5.74
Tanganyika					−0.70[b]	−1.26
Sweden	−2.60	−1.45	0.90	0.82		−3.52
U.S.A.	0.52	0.08	0.04	1.83	1.95	7.52

* Taken from Schull and Neel (1965, p. 347).
a Includes neonatal deaths.
b Inclusion of stillbirths uncertain.
c Includes stillbirths.

observations from France, the *B/A* ratios are small—10 or less. It will be recalled that under the Morton-Crow-Muller formulation the ratio of the inbred to the random load provides crucial evidence with respect to the contributions of mutation and selection to the concealed variability in a population only if this ratio is large, and then only if gene action is, in general, non-synergistic. These studies do not reveal ratios which may be construed as unambiguously supporting the view that the load revealed by inbreeding is mainly of the mutational variety. The observed values are, in fact, consistent with a substantial portion of the load being segregational in origin.

Again, with singular exceptions, there is some agreement in the probable number of lethal equivalents, particularly at those stages of development, such as stillbirths and neonatal deaths, for which the studies are most comparable. We note, for example, that relatively fewer lethal genes appear to manifest themselves as stillbirths or deaths in the first month of life than at subsequent ages. It is also of interest that the variation in the estimates derived from a single area in, for example, France or Japan, nearly equals the variation from one area of the world to another. Alternatively stated, there seems to be as much intra-area variation as inter-areas variation. With regard to miscarriages and deaths after the neonatal period, interpretations of the data must be more guarded. Thus, it is difficult to ascertain whether a major portion of lethal genes are or are not manifest in early zygotic mortality because of the apparent heterogeneity between the four studies (estimates range from —2.60 to 3.20) and the admitted difficulty in obtaining reliable information on losses at this stage of life. . . . As to infantile and juvenile deaths, the differences which exist between the studies in number of years at risk of death preclude sweeping generalizations. This fact notwithstanding, it seems unlikely that the mean number of lethal equivalents acting after parturition, and more especially after the first month of life, is apt to exceed 3. The biological, psychological, and sociological impact of these genes upon a community or population is, as we have seen, presently beyond assessment.

Genetic Load in Drosophila

I would like to discuss some important findings from other organisms, and then relate them to the problem in man. The most suitable organism for this subject has been the fruit fly (*Drosophila*). Unlike human beings, fruit flies are easily handled experimentally. Using cytological techniques, they can be made completely homozygous for one or more pairs of chromosomes. It is also possible to collect a large number of flies from a natural population, to breed flies which carry lethal free chromosomes, and so on. And experiments can be done with a high degree of accuracy. With these advantages the fruit fly data have revealed several features, for which no equivalent human information is available.

One feature is the distribution of various viability classes of genes, in equilibrium natural populations, measured for homozygotes. They vary from lethals to normal genes. In all the *Drosophila* species examined, the distribution, or prevalence, of viability classes in homozygotes is bimodal. One case is presented in Figure 1. One frequency peak lies just below the average normal viability (1.0); this must mean that in natural populations there are many deleterious genes with rather weak effects, bordering closely on the normal. The second peak of the distribution lies at the level of complete lethality. Therefore two quite distinct classes of genes are found, with intermediate classes being much less frequent. The two main classes are easily distinguished, hence the loads due these classes can also be distinguished. Making flies homozygous for chromosomes from an equilibrium population, and comparing the viability of these flies to that of flies possessing pairs of randomly chosen chromosomes, we can measure the inbred load. If lethal carrying chromosomes are excluded in such an experiment, the result reveals the load due to the class of mildly deleterious genes, and inclusion of lethals reveals the total inbred load. Greenberg and Crow (1960) made one of the first attempts to evaluate these loads. The result of their experiment using the second chromosome of *Drosophila melanogaster* is summarized in Table 2.

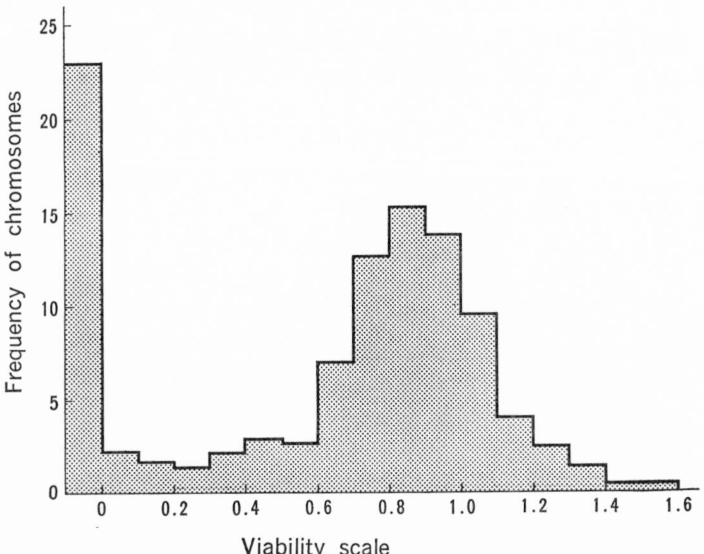

FIG. 1. Distribution of frequencies of viability (from Greenberg and Crow, 1960).

TABLE 2. Genetic load, expressed in lethal equivalents, for the second chromosome in equilibrium populations of *D. melanogaster* (from Greenburg and Crow, 1960).

Population	Number of chromosomes tested	Load due to detrimental (not lethal) genes	Load due to lethal genes	Total
Madison*	231	0.235±0.029	0.300±0.051	0.536±0.049
Cage population (a)**	121	0.185±0.034	0.272±0.066	0.457±0.061
Cage population (b)**	113	0.136±0.029	0.271±0.063	0.406±0.060
Weighted mean	465	0.180±0.017	0.287±0.034	0.467±0.032

* A wild population collected in Madison, Wisconsin.

** Maintained as a large population for several years by Dr. Bruce Wallace.

From the data in Table 2 we can conclude that on average the typical second chromosome in these flies carries 0.47 lethal equivalents, of which 0.29 are lethals and 0.18 are non-lethal detrimentals, in comparison with the average heterozygote viability in the population. (According to the above definition of the genetic load, the lethal equivalent has to be calculated in relation to the most fit genotype, and this correction is made in the later discussions.) Since the second chromosome of *Drosophila melanogaster* constitutes about 40 percent of the total genome, a linear extrapolation gives an estimate of about 1.2 lethal equivalents per genome. There are a number of experiments using several species of *Drosophila*, from which, though rather indirectly, the inbred loads can be estimated. A summary of such calculations is given in Greenberg and Crow (1960); the values of the total load vary around a mean value 0.55, while the ratios of the detrimental load to the lethal load vary around a mean 1.1.

The degree of gene interaction is one of our interests in this symposium. *Drosophila* data can provide useful information on the average interaction between detrimental genes at different chromosomes and at different loci. The degree of the interaction can be measured by comparing the amount of viability depression from making the second (or the third) chromosome homozygous with the depression due to homozygosity for both the second and third chromosomes. That is, if the detrimental genes act independently, then the average viability of flies homozygous for both the second and third chromosomes should be equal to the product of the viability of flies homozygous for the second chromosome alone and that of flies homozygous for the third chromosome alone. Any deviation in the viability from the product is a measure of the interaction between the genes on the different chromosomes. A similar comparison of viability depression result-

TABLE 3. Viability expressed when the second and/or the third chromosomes are made completely homozygous ($f=1$).

Species (*Drosophila*)	Second chromosome	Third chromosome	Interaction (I)	Author
melanogaster	0.91	0.88	0.97	Temin *et al.* (1969)
pseudoobscura	0.89	0.86	0.88	Spassky *et al.* (1965)
melanogaster	0.95	0.85	0.92	Kosuda (1971)

ing from different degrees of inbreeding on a particular chromosome enables us to infer the interaction of genes at different loci on the same chromosome. Some data for the average interaction of the genes on the second and third chromosomes of two *Drosophila* species are given in Table 3. In the table, the index I is the ratio of the observed viability of flies homozygous for the two chromosomes to that expected from the product of the two. If there is no interaction, I should be equal to 1, and if the interaction is strongly synergistic, I becomes small. From the table, we can say that there is a slight interaction, but it is not very strong. Studies on the interaction among different loci on the same chromosome lead to a similar conclusion.

The spontaneous mutation rate of lethal genes in *Drosophila* is about 0.015 per gamete per generation. This is based mainly on experiments in which a lethal-free chromosome is kept heterozygous with minimally possible selection for several generations, during which mutations accumulate and are later detected by making the chromosome homozygous. This value of the mutation rate 0.015/gamete/generation is reliable. Experiments of this type can reveal the accumulated effect of viability-reducing mutants. This is a class of mutants of which our knowledge for man is very limited, and we can only make an extrapolation from *Drosophila* data. A number of large-scale reliable experiments concerning mildly deleterious mutants were conducted by T. Mukai and his colleagues during the last 15 years, and the nature of this mutant class in *Drosophila* came to be well understood. The first of Mukai's major findings was that the homozygous load caused by such mildly deleterious mutations accumulated at a rate of about 0.004 per generation. This is shown graphically in Figure 2 for about 60 generations of accumulation, and was tested at various stages by making the flies homozygous (Mukai, 1964). This is the accumulation rate per chromosome, and since the second chromosome of *Drosophila melanogaster* constitutes about 40 percent of the total genome, the rate per gamete is about 0.01 per generation.

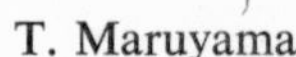

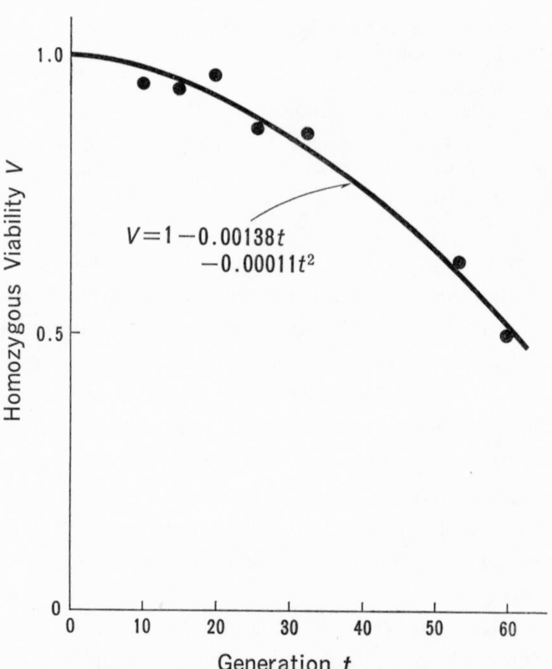

FIG. 2. The relationship between homozygous viability and the number of generations for the accumulation of mildly detrimental mutants, in the second chromosome of *Drosophila melanogaster* (from Mukai, 1969).

Even from this data alone, without further argument, it seems apparent that accumulation of mutations really occurs when the selection is relaxed. This may be happening in human populations with the advancement of medicine and of technology. In the case of *Drosophila*, after about 60 generations, mildly detrimental mutants had accumulated to such an extent that the viability of homozygotes was reduced to 50 percent of the original. In these experiments, lethal genes were excluded, and the tests were conducted only with mildly deleterious mutants.

Translating this load into an actual mutation rate is an uncertain proposition because there is always the possibility of a large number of mutants with nearly zero effect. Any estimate is therefore necessarily minimal. From the variance among replicate lines, the mutation rate of mildly deleterious mutants is estimated to be at least 10 times as high as lethals, more likely 20 times. Summarizing:

Mildly deleterious mutants/generation	Lethals/generation
$\Sigma u_i s_i = 0.004$ (load)	
$\bar{s} = 0.038$	
Σu_i (mutation rate) $= 0.177$/chromosome (2)	$\Sigma v_i = 0.006$/chromosome (2)
Σu_i (mutation rate) $= 0.442$/gamete	$\Sigma v_i = 0.015$/gamete

where u_i is the rate of mutation of a mutant of effect s_i, and $\bar{s}$ is the mean of s_i, and v_i is the lethal mutation rate at locus i, (see Mukai, 1964; Mukai, 1968; Mukai *et al.*, 1972).

I would like to emphasize that the rate of mutation for mildly deleterious mutants is very much higher than that for lethals. Therefore if man is like *Drosophila* with respect to the rate of mildly deleterious mutations, and if the Haldane-Muller principle applies, then the expressed mutational load due to mild mutants can be much higher than that due to strongly harmful mutants and lethal genes. It is possible that 10 or 20 times more selection is operating on the mildly deleterious mutants than on lethal mutants.

From the data given by Schull and Neel (1965), Mukai has calculated the random load and the inbred load in man, and has partitioned the load into the part due to lethals and the part due to mild genes (assuming that the ratios of the two components are the same in man and *Drosophila*). The following summary was adapted from Mukai (1975), where he gives a lucid account on the genetic load in man and *Drosophila*:

		Inbred load/gamete (equilibrium)		Mutation rate/gamete	
		Man	*Drosophila*	Man	*Drosophila*
Total		1.6	2.2	0.2	0.3∼0.4
Partitioned	Mildly delet.	0.8	1.1	0.19	0.3∼0.4
	Lethal	0.8	1.1	0.01	0.013

Mukai *et al.* (1972) revealed another feature of the *Drosophila* data for which no equivalent human information is available. They made an attempt to infer the persistence time of mutant genes by comparing the mildly detrimental load in newly arising mutants with that in a population at equilibrium. The relevant information for the second chromosome in *Drosophila melanogaster* is as follows:

	Homozygous load/chrom. 2		
	New Mutants/ generation	Natural population (equilibrium)	Ratio, average persistence time (generations)
Mild	0.004	0.30	74
Lethal	0.006	0.50	84

The striking fact is that the ratios for the two cases are about the same. The ratio is the mean persistence time of mutant genes; therefore, despite the fact that mildly deleterious genes and lethal genes are very different in their homozygous effects, they persist approximately the same number of generations in the population before they are eliminated by selection. We may expect the mild mutants to persist many times longer and therefore to have higher ratios. But the experimental result is contrary to this expectation: both classes of mutants appear to persist about the same number of generations. Neither inbreeding nor homozygous elimination is sufficient, so there must be a large amount of selection against heterozygotes.

These findings from *Drosophila* can be summarized as follows:

(1) Inbred load:
Mild mutants≈Lethals

(2) Persistence time:
Mild mutants≈Lethals (Selection against heterozygotes)

(3) Mutation rate:
Mild mutants≫Lethals

(4) Expressed load (Random load):
Mild mutants≫Lethals (probably)

Mukai and Yamazaki (1964, 1968) provided more direct evidence that the average degree of newly arising mildly derimental mutants is as high as 0.4, which is far higher than that of lethals. If man is like *Drosophila*, a major share of the expressed mutation load is through selection against heterozygotes. Therefore even recessive mutants hardly ever become homozygous in large populations, but exert their impact on the population through heterozygous effect.

If the relatively large heterozygous effect is also true in mammals, an increased mutation rate should have an effect on the fitness of immediately following generations through the heterozygous effects of many mildly detrimental mutants. However, attempts to measure the effects of presumptive new mutations on fitness and other traits of heterozygotes, either after one generation of parental exposure or after several generations in which the mutations may accumulate, have, in general, been unsuccessful in mice experiments (see Green, 1968). High dose treatment with EMS in *Drosophila* has produced about 5 percent heterozygous depression of viability, but in this case the fitness reduction can be entirely accounted for by heterozygous effect of lethals (Ohnishi, 1976). Therefore a strong experimental basis for a large immediate effect of an enhanced mutation rate is not clear, and the way in which the mildly detrimental genes and lethals are eliminated from the population remains still uncertain. Thus the way in which the effect of these mutants can be translated into terms of human welfare is not evident. This is one of our problems for the future in human genetics.

Relaxed Selection

Following Crow (1972, 1974), I should like to discuss briefly some of the obvious consequences of the relaxed selection which has been brought to our human society. For simplicity, assume that a previously fatal disease has become completely curable by medical treatment. I wish to examine the consequences in two hypothetical situations. First, assume that the disease is caused by a dominant lethal. Then, before the successful treatment became possible, every case of the disease was the result of a mutation which occurred in that generation, because no dominant lethal genes are transmitted. But with successful treatment, every new mutant will now survive, and the incidence of this disease will increase proportionally. Therefore the disease incidence will be doubled in one generation, tripled in two generations, quadrupled in three generations, and so forth. The increase, in the case of dominant mutants, is very rapid. The situation is quite different, however, when the disease is caused by a recessive lethal gene. The lethal genes added to the next generation as a result of the medical treatment would be from homozygotes with frequency p^2, where p is the present gene frequency. The gene frequency in the next generation would be

$$p' = p + p^2 = p(1 + p).$$

Therefore the proportion of the recessive homozygotes for this gene would be

$$(p')^2 = p^2(1+p)^2$$

and the increment in the recessive homozygotes,

$$\Delta(p^2) = \frac{(p')^2 - p^2}{p^2} = \frac{p^2 + 2p^3 + p^4 - p^2}{p^2} = 2p + p^2.$$

If p is small, the increment in the incidence of this disease is small. For example, if $p=0.01$, then the increase is only 2 percent, and it may take about 35 generations to double the present incidence of the disease. Obviously, such an increase is very slow and probably is not a matter of great immediate concern. Crow (1972) says:

> With genetic counselling a person with a dominant disease will know the 50 percent risk for each child and can make a rational decision based on whether his own life has been miserable or fulfilling. The burden for future generations can be calculated in terms of the cost of the treatment. For the recessive disease the increase is too small to worry about in the near future.

In the above argument we assumed that the treatment was complete, but it is also possible to proceed with the discussion under a more realistic assumption. See Holloway and Smith (1975).

This is, however, only one aspect of the problem. Other practical questions might be how the relaxation of selection can be measured and what the implications are. Matsunaga (1966) and Crow (1972) present lucid discussions on these subjects. They were concerned with the measurement of selection intensity and its trends in human populations. Using a method which measures an upper limit of selection intensity or selection opportunity, Matsunaga has shown, from Japanese census reports, that as a consequence of family planning and of childhood mortality reduction the intensity or opportunity of selection had steadily declined in Japan during the 1950s and early 1960s. There is no doubt that the same tendency must be continuing. Crow (1972) has reported a similar result using U. S. Census data. Since these analyses do not include the large portion of genetic selection which might be taking place through embryonic deaths, it is not possible to conclude that all genetic selection ceases to exist, but nevertheless these represent a real decline in the intensity or opportunity of selection.

Some Remarks on the Theory of Genetic Load

Because of the nature of this symposium, I have talked mainly about empirical aspects of genetic load, particularly about the mutational load in man and *Drosophila*, to which much of the available data refers. I should like, however, to call the reader's attention to the existence of a vast number of sophisticated theoretical studies on the subject. One may refer to Kimura (1960) and Crow (1970), who give very comprehensive reviews of the theory of genetic load. These two reviews, by two leaders in the advancement of the theory of genetic load, present probably the most thorough accounts of the theory up to 1960 and 1970, respectively. There are numerous other reviews and discussions of the concept and theory of genetic load: Crow, 1958, 1963, 1968; Crow and Kimura, 1963; Kimura, 1960a. Some aspects of the genetic load theory have been questioned conceptually, particularly those which do not lower the average fitness of the population in comparison with the hypothetical situation in which the factor under consideration is absent (Wallace, 1968, 1970).

It is also worth noting that some of the topical problems in genetics and evolution theory have arisen from considerations of the genetic load. When Kimura (1968) put forward the neutral hypothesis of molecular evolution, as observed among homologous proteins in different species diverging from a common origin, his argument was based on substitutional load—that is, on the fact that the observed rate of gene substitution is too high to be supported by the load allocable to this process. Basing their calculation on a probable amount of tolerance of the mutation load in man and on an estimated rate of detrimental mutation in mammalian genes, Ohta and Kimura (1971) have concluded that the total number of (informational or functional) genes in man is about 30,000—about 6 percent of the total DNA, which consists of about 3×10^9 nucleotide pairs. See also Muller (1967).

Summary

The words "genetic load" and "load of mutation" were first used by Muller (1950) in an attempt to assess the impact of the dangers of human hereditary defects. Many human diseases have a genetic basis, and these ills constitute a burden not only to afflicted persons but also to society as a whole in the sense that they create a major public health problem. In regard to the genetic load caused by detrimental mutants (the mutation load), a powerful principle states that the impact of mutation on the average fitness of the population is equal to the mutation rate and is independent of the effect of the individual mutant on fitness (Haldane, 1937; Muller, 1950).

The concept of genetic loads has been generalized by Crow (1958) to measure the amount of selection associated with certain genetic variability maintained in a population. In this sense, the genetic load can be classified according to its cause, and it is not necessarily a burden or bad; it is often the price paid by a species for evolution.

Morton, Crow, and Muller (1956) developed a general method to evaluate, in terms of lethal equivalents, the inbred load which would be expressed if the population were made complete homozygous ($f=1$). In theory, this method also enables us to infer the nature of the homozygous load concealed in the heterozygous condition. Although the data on human inbreeding effects have not been very reproducible, it is estimated that the average human individual might carry at least one, and probably several, hidden lethal equivalents (Schull and Neel, 1965, and others).

In *Drosophila*, where the measures are precise and reproducible, there are about two lethal equivalents per fly. About half of the viability depression from inbreeding is attributable to monogenic lethals; the other half is the cumulative effect of a much large number of genes with individually small effects (Greenberg and Crow, 1960; Temin, 1966; Kosuda, 1971; Mukai and Yamaguchi, 1974; Mukai, 1976). In *Drosophila*, the lethal mutation rate per gamete per generation is about 0.015, but, strikingly, the rate of mildly detrimental mutants is estimated to be about 0.4 (Mukai, 1964; Mukai *et al.*, 1972), which is much higher than the lethal mutation rate. From comparison of the mildly detrimental load in newly arising mutants to that in a population at equilibrium and from an analogous comparison for lethals, it is concluded that despite a large difference in their homozygous effects (lethal or mild), mutants of either class persist about the same number of generations ($70 \sim 80$) in the population before they are eliminated by selection (Mukai *et al.*, 1972). Therefore the mild mutants are eliminated from the population at rates comparable to those for lethals. Neither inbreeding nor homozygote elimination is sufficient, hence most of selection in either class must be operating against heterozygotes: the degree of dominance in the mild mutants is high, probably about 0.4.

The results of work by Mukai and his associates, together with the Haldane-Muller principle, have very important implications for the human welfare problem. If the results from *Drosophila* can be applied to man, a major part of the expressed mutation load is due to the heterozygous effect of mildly detrimental mutants.

Acknowledgements

I wish to thank Drs. E. Inouye, M. Kimura, E. Matsunaga, the executive committee of the symposium, and the Japan Medical Research Foundation for giving me the opportunity to speak on this subject at the symposium and for their valuable aid. Drs. E. Matsunaga and T. Mukai have kindly read the manuscript, and I owe to them a number of substantial improvements. Also I would like to thank Drs. S. Ishiwa, C. Smith, and Y. Yamada, who have offered advice and suggestions.

REFERENCES

Arner, G. B. L. 1908. Consanguineous marriage in the American population. *Columbia Univ. Studies Hist. Econ. Public. Law* **31**: 1–99.

Cavalli-Sforza, L. L., and Bodmer, W. F. 1971. *The genetics of human populations*. Freeman, San Francisco, U.S.A.

Crow, J. F. 1958. Some possibilities for measuring selection intensities in man. *Hum. Biol.* **30**: 1–12.

Crow, J. F. 1963. The concept of genetic load: A reply. *Am. J. Hum. Genet.* **15**: 310–315.

Crow, J. F. 1968. The cost of evolution and genetic loads. *In* Dronamraju, K. (Ed.), *Haldane and modern biology*, pp. 165–178. Johns Hopkins Press, Baltimore, U.S.A.

Crow, J. F. 1970. Genetic loads and the cost of natural selection. *In* Kojima, K. (Ed.), *Mathematical topics in population genetics*. Springer-Verlag, Berlin-Heidelberg-New York.

Crow, J. F. 1972. Some effects of relaxed selection and mutation. *Proc. 4th Int. Cong. Hum. Genet.* 155–166.

Crow, J. F. 1973. Population perspective. *In* Hilton, B., Callahan, D., Harris, M., Condliffe, P., and Berkley, B. (Eds.), *Ethical issues in human genetics*. Plenum, New York, U.S.A.

Crow, J. F. 1974. Mutation, selection and man's future. *In* Kimura, M. (Ed.), *Future of man* (in Japanese). Baifukan, Tokyo, Japan.

Crow, J. F., and Kimura, M. 1964. The theory of genetic loads. *Genetics Today: Proc. XI Int. Cong. Genet.* Pergamon Press, Oxford, England.

Crow, J. F., and Morton, N. E. 1960. The genetic load due to mother-child incompatibility. *Amer. Naturalist* **94**: 413–419.

Dobzhansky, Th. 1955. A review of some fundamental concepts and problems of population genetics. *Cold Spring Harb. Symp. Quant. Biol.* **20**: 1–15.

Dobzhansky, Th. 1957. Genetic loads in natural populations. *Science* **126**: 191–194.

Felsenstein, J. 1971. On the biological significance of the cost of gene substitution. *Amer. Naturalist* **105**: 1–11.

Green, E. L. 1968. Genetic effects of radiation on mammalian populations. *Annual Review of Genetics* **2**: 87–120.

Greenberg, R., and Crow, J. F. 1960. A comparison of the lethal effect of lethal and detrimental chromosomes from *Drosophila populations. Genetics* **45**: 1154–1168.

Haldane, J. B. S. 1937. The effect of variation on fitness. *Amer. Naturalist* **71**: 337–349.

Haldane, J. B. S. 1957. The cost of natural selection. *J. Genet.* **55**: 511–524.

Hiraizumi, Y., and Crow, J. F. 1960. Heterozygous effects on viability, fertility, rate of development, and longevity of *Drosophila* chromosomes that are lethal when homozygous. *Genetics* **45**: 1071–1083.

Holloway, S. M., and Smith, C. 1975. Effects of various medical and social practices on the frequency of genetic disorders. *Amer. J. Human Genet.* **27**: 614–627.

Kimura, M. 1960. Genetic load of a population and its significance in evolution (in Japanese). *Japan. J. Genet.* **35**: 7–33.

Kimura, M. 1960a. *Population genetics* (in Japanese). Baifukan, Tokyo, Japan.

Kimura, M. 1961. Some calculations on the mutational load. *Japan. J. Genet.* **36** suppl: 179–190.

Kimura, M. 1968. Evolutionary rate at the molecular level. *Nature* **217**: 624–626.

Kimura, M., Maruyama, T., and Crow, J. F. 1963. The mutation load in small populations. *Genetics* **48**: 1303–1312.

Kimura, M., and Maruyama, T. 1969. The substitutional load in a finite population. *Heredity* **24**: 101–114.

Kimura, M., and Ohta, T. 1970. Genetic loads at a polymorphic locus which is maintained by frequency dependent selection. *Genet. Res.* **16**: 145–150.

Kosuda, K. 1971. Synergistic interaction between second and third chromosomes on viability of *Drosophila melanogaster. Jap. J. Genet.* **46**: 41–52.

Matsunaga, E. 1966. Possible genetic consequences of family planning. *J. Am. Med. Assoc.* **198**: 533–540.

McKusick, V. A. 1975. *Mendelian inheritance in man.* Johns Hopkins Press, Baltimore, U.S.A.

Morton, N. E. 1960. The mutational load due to detrimental genes in man. *Am. J. Hum. Genet.* **12**: 348–364.

Morton, N. E. 1961. Morbidity of children from consanguineous marriages. *In* Steinberg, A. (Ed.), *Progress in medical genetics*, vol. 1: 261–291. Grune and Stratton, New York, U.S.A.

Morton, N. E., Crow, J. F., and Muller, H. J. 1956. An estimate of the mutational damage in man from data on consanguineous marriages. *Proc. Natl. Acad. Sci. U. S. A.* **42**: 855–863.

Mukai, T. 1964. The genetic structure of natural populations of *Drosophila melanogaster*. I. Spontaneous mutation rate of polygenes controlling viability. *Genetics* **50**: 1–19.

Mukai, T. 1968. Experimental studies on the mechanism involved in the maintenance of genetic variability in *Drosophila* populations (in Japanese). *Japan. J. Genet.* 399–413.

Mukai, T. 1969. Maintenance of polygenic and isoallelic variation in populations. *Proc. XII Int. Cong. Genet.* vol. **3**: 293–308.

Mukai, T. 1975. Dynamics of mutants in populations. (in Japanese). *In* Kimura, M. (Ed.), *Foundation of human genetics*, Iwanami Modern Biology Series vol. 6. Iwanami, Tokyo, Japan.

Mukai, T. 1976. Unpublished.

Mukai, T., Cardellino, R. A., Watanabe, T. K., and Crow, J. F. 1974. The genetic variance for viability and its components in a local population of *Drosophila melanogaster*. *Genetics* **78**: 1195–1208.

Mukai, T., Chigusa, S. I., Mettler, L. E., and Crow, J. F. 1972. Mutation rate and dominance of genes affecting viability in *Drosophila melanogaster*. *Genetics* **72**: 335–355.

Mukai, T., and Yamaguchi, O. 1974. The genetic structure of natural populations of *Drosophila melanogaster*. XI. Genetic variability in a local population. *Genetics* **76**: 339–366.

Mukai, T., and Yamazaki, T. 1964. Position effect of spontaneous mutant polygenes controlling viability in *Drosophila melanogaster*. *Proc. Japan Acad.* **40**: 840–845.

Mukai, T., and Yamazaki, T. 1968. The genetic structure of natural populations of *Drosophila melanogaster*. V. Coupling-repulsion effect of spontaneous mutant polygenes controlling viability. *Genetics* **59**: 513–535.

Muller, H. J. 1948. Mutation prophylaxis. *Bull. N.Y. Acad. Med.* **24**: 447–469.

Muller, H. J. 1950. Our load of mutations. *Am. J. Hum. Genet.* **2**: 111–176.

Muller, H. J. 1956. Further studies bearing on the load of mutations in man. *Acta Genet. Stat. Med.* **6**: 157–168.

Muller, H. J. 1967. The gene material as the initiator and the organizing basis. *In* Brink, R. A. (Ed.), *Heritage from Mendel.* The University of Wisconsin Press, Madison, Wis., U.S.A.

Ohnishi, O. 1976. Spontaneous and methansulfonate induced mutations controlling viability in *Drosophila melanogaster*. III. Heterozygous effect of polygenic mutations. To appear.

Ohta, T., and Kimura, M. 1971. Functional organization of genetic material as a product of molecular evolution. *Nature* **233**: 118–119.

Penrose, L. S. 1957. A note on the prevalence of genes for deleterious recessive traits in man. *Ann. Hum. Genet.* **21**: 222–223.

Reed, S. C. 1954. A test for heterozygous deleterious recessives. *J. Hered.* **45**: 17–18.

Russell, W. L. 1952. Mammalian radiation genetics. In J. J. Nickson (Ed.), *Symposium on radiobiology*, pp. 427–440. John Wiley and Sons, New York, U.S.A.

Schull, W. J., and Neel, J. V. 1965. *The effect of inbreeding on Japanese children*, pp. 328–351. Harper and Row, New York, U.S.A.

Slatis, H. M. 1954. A method of estimating the frequency of abnormal recessive genes in man. *Am. J. Hum. Genet.* **6**: 412–418.

Spassky, B., Dobzhansky, Th., and Anderson, W. W. 1965. Genetics of natural populations. XXXVI. Epistatic interaction of the components of the genetic load in *Drosophila pseudoobscura*. *Genetics* **52**: 653–664.

Temin, R. G., Meyer, H. U., Dawson, P. S., and Crow, J. F. 1969. The influence of epistasis on homozygous viability depression in *Drosophila melanogaster*. *Genetics* **61**: 497–519.

Wallace, B. 1968. *Topics in population genetics*. Norton, New York, U.S.A.

Wallace, B. 1970. *Genetic load: Its biological and conceptual aspects*. Prentice-Hall, New Jersey, U.S.A.

DISCUSSION

Possible Genetic Consequences of Relaxed Selection against Common Disorders with Complex Inheritance

Ei Matsunaga

Dr. Maruyama has reviewed some obvious consequences of relaxed selection against autosomal dominant and recessive diseases. I should like to focus the discussion on the case of common disorders with complex inheritance.

Common disorders with relatively high heritability make up a major portion of our genetic burden in terms of social cost involved in treatment, cure, and rehabilitation. With increasing success in medical treatment for many of those disorders, it is expected that the incidence of patients requiring treatment will gradually rise from generation to generation, and so our genetic burden will be increased in the future. While this is theoretically true for a long-range future, relatively little study has been made to evaluate the magnitude of this effect. Some years ago a WHO Scientific Group (1972) reported that the restoration of full fertility to all of the patients would result in a 3–5 percent increase in the traits per generation, or a doubling time of 14–23 generations. Recently, Holloway and Smith (1975) noted that the maximum increase in incidence due to improved fitness of affected individuals is likely to be about 5 percent per generation. I have examined this problem using empirical figures and found that the increase is not likely to be by compound interest, at least over the next few generations, with which we are mostly concerned (Matsunaga, 1976). In the following discussion, it is assumed that there is no change in the environmental factors contributing to the disease; no assumption is made, however, about possible mechanisms maintaining harmful genes for the condition that are produced by recurrent mutations.

Let P_0 be the frequency at birth of an abnormality that has been lethal until an efficient medical treatment was discovered. In order to consider the maximum possible effect of relaxed selection, let us assume that the condition in all the patients is from now on completely repaired. Let x be the proportion of affected children born to normal parents, y the propor-

Department of Human Genetics, National Institute of Genetics, Mishima, Japan.

tion of affected born to repaired patients with normal spouses, and z the proportion of affected children when both parents have been repaired ($1 \geqq z > y > x > 0$). By definition, $P_0 = x$. Under random mating, the frequency of the abnormality in the next generation, P_1, will be:

$$P_1 = (1 - P_0)^2 x + 2P_0(1 - P_0)y + P_0{}^2 z.$$

As to individuals with normal phenotypes, two groups may now be distinguished: Group 1 having normal parents with a frequency of $N_{1.1} = (1 - P_0)^2\ (1 - x)$, and Group 2, having at least one parent affected and repaired, with a frequency of $N_{1.2} = 1 - P_1 - N_{1.1}$. Since the genetic predisposition to the abnormality of Group 2 individuals must be, on the average, somewhat higher than that of Group 1 individuals, let u, v, and w be the proportions of affected children born to the matings of Group $1 \times$ Group 2, Group $2 \times$ Group 2, and Group $2 \times$ affected individuals, respectively ($z > w > y > v > u > x$). If y and z remain the same, the frequency of the trait in the second generation, P_2, will be:

$$P_2 = N_{1.1}{}^2 x + 2N_{1.1}N_{1.2}u + N_{1.2}{}^2 v + 2N_{1.1}P_1 y + 2N_{1.2}P_1 w + P_1{}^2 z.$$

If x, y, z, u, v, and w remain unchanged from generation to generation, it is possible to calculate by the same procedure the frequency of the trait in the third and subsequent generations.

Taking as an example congenital heart disease, not including those cases involved in single-gene or chromosomal syndromes, x and y have been estimated to be about 0.004 and 0.04, respectively (Carter, 1969; Emery, 1974), while no empirical figures are available for other parameters. However, applying Falconer's procedure (Falconer, 1965) to the observed values of x and y, the heritability may be estimated as about 60 percent which in turn may provide the basis for estimating z to be probably of the order of 0.2–0.4, and u, v, and w being about 0.008, 0.015, and 0.07 respectively. The wider range of z does not affect the result much, because the chance of marriage between patients both of whom were repaired could be very small. The same argument may also apply to v and w. Table 1 illustrates the increase in the relative incidence in the next few generations for $x = 0.004$, $y = 0.04$, and $u = 0.008$ and for two differing values of z, v and w, assuming that all cases of congenital heart disease were completely repaired. It is interesting to note that the increment is the greatest in the first generation and becomes smaller and smaller until there will be practically no more increase after six generations; the overall increase in the trait frequency will

TABLE 1. Numerical illustration of the maximum possible increase in relative incidence of congenital heart disease, with $x=0.004$, $y=0.04$ and $u=0.008$, in the next few generations (Matsunaga, 1976).

Generation	Relative incidence	
	$v=0.015$, $w=0.07$, $z=0.2$	$v=0.03$, $w=0.10$, $z=0.4$
0	1.00000	1.00000
1	1.07250	1.07330
2	1.09359	1.09527
3	1.09628	1.09816
4	1.09681	1.09874
5	1.09689	1.09884
6	1.09691	1.09885
7	1.09691	1.09885

be at most about 10 percent, as the values for z, v, and w vary to some extent.

However, the above conclusion should be taken with some reservations, because of the over-simplified calculations. First, I have assumed that the proportion of affected born to normal individuals whose parents were normal remains unchanged from generation to generation, without regard to the status of their grandparents or more remote ancestors. Second, I have assumed that the proportion of affected born to affected individuals remains the same, whether their parents were affected or not. Obviously, these two assumptions do not hold on the basis of polygenic inheritance with threshold. The genetic predisposition of phenotypically normal individuals having normal parents must be, on the average, slightly greater if, for example, their grandparents were affected than if none of them were affected. Likewise, the genetic predisposition of affected individuals must be greater, on the average, if one of their parents was affected than if neither of them was affected, and still greater if both parents were affected. Consequently, with increasing frequency of normal or affected individuals having affected ancestors, the values of the above six parameters would begin to rise gradually. However, because of rare occurrence of affected individuals having affected parents, the effect of changing x only may be of relative importance in the near future. I have studied this point in some detail, and found that there would be an additional increase in the frequency of the trait by about 1 percent or less in the third generation, less than that in the fourth generation, and so on. Thus a slightly greater increment than was shown in the table would take place in the frequency of the trait after the third generation, but the discrepancy could be minor as far as the next few generations are concerned. It should be noted that with the passage of generations the discrepancy will become gradually greater and greater, though a number of generations will be required until the extent of the increment in the frequency of the trait attains a noticeable level.

In conclusion, the expected rise in our genetic burden due to complete relaxation of selection against common disorders with complex inheritance will be, as far as the near future is concerned, such that the maximum possible increment will take place in the first generation, with additional increment rapidly diminishing with subsequent generations. For congenital heart disease, for example, the restoration of full fertility to all of the patients will incur an increase in the frequency of the disease at birth by about 10 percent after five to ten generations.

REFERENCES

Carter, C. O. 1969. Genetics of common disorders. *Brit. Med. Bull.* **25**: 52–57.

Emery, A. E. H. 1974. *Elements of Medical Genetics*, third ed., p. 200. Churchill Livingston, Edinburgh—London, England.

Falconer, D. S. 1965. The inheritance of liability to certain diseases, estimated from the incidence among relatives. *Ann. Human Genet.* **29**: 51–76.

Holloway, S. M. and Smith, C. 1975. Effects of various medical and social practices on the frequency of genetic disorders. *Am. J. Human Genet.* **27**: 614–627.

Matsunaga, E. 1976. Possible genetic consequences of relaxed selection against common disorders with complex inheritance. *Hum. Genet.* **31**: 53–57.

WHO Scientific Group. 1965. Genetic disorders: Prevention, treatment and rehabilitation. *WHO Techn. Rep. Ser.* No. 497, p. 33 and 45.

II GENETIC AND ENVIRONMENTAL FACTORS IN COMMON DISEASES

Genetic and Environmental Factors in Congenital Heart Disease

Masahiko Ando, Atsuyoshi Takao, and Katsuhiko Mori

It is self-evident that the ideal management of congenital heart malformations should be prevention. Most congenital anomalies of the heart are probably a result of complex interactions between genetic predispositions and environmental factors; this is a specific mode of inheritance, called multifactorial inheritance with threshold (Falconer, 1960; Nora, 1968). Single gene disorders and chromosomal syndromes appear to account for a small percentage of cases. Therefore, the better the genetic predispositions and environmental triggers are identified, the greater will be the chance to reduce the incidence of congenital heart disease (CHD).

At the present time, the multifactorial model is still a hypothetical theory, and the exact natures of genetic predispositions and environmental teratogens are not yet known. Accordingly, several preliminary studies were conducted to search for the nature of the two factors, based upon data from Japanese patients with established diagnoses of cardiac defects (Ando, 1969; Mori, 1973; Ando, 1973; Ando, 1975a).

Multifactorial Model for Congenital Heart Disease

The evidences for multifactorial inheritance are entirely indirect, and are based upon incidence in the general population and familial recurrence of paticular anomalies. To demonstrate this theoretical model, family studies were performed in common congenital heart diseases (Ando, 1969; Mori, 1973).

Frequency of cardiac anomalies in first relatives. Empiric recurrence risks of 13 common heart lesions in siblings of an affected individual, when the parents are normal, are shown in Table 1 and compared with the

The Heart Institute of Japan, Tokyo Women's Medical College, Tokyo, Japan.

TABLE 1. Observed and expected recurrence risks in siblings. General population incidence was estimated as 0.7 percent (Neel, 1958). As the population incidences for each category of the cardiac anomalies are not available for Japanese, relative frequency of the defects in patients admitted during 1969 was substituted; this is shown in Figure 1. Siblings with known congenital heart disease were incorporated as proband cases only when they were admitted to our hospital for cardiovascular diagnosis; therefore, the observed values may be slightly underestimated for some of the defects.

Anomalies	Probands	Affected Siblings		Expected($\sqrt{p}$
		No.	(%)	
VSD	1241	18/1237	(1.46)	4.9
ASDII	557	13/1110	(1.17)	3.2
TOF	296	6/380	(1.58)	3.6
PDA	295	8/408	(1.96)	2.7
PS	123	3/199	(1.51)	1.5
TGA, DORV	153	3/171	(1.75)	1.3
ECD	80	2/103	(1.94)	1.3
APVD	41	2/45	(4.44)	1.3
Dextro., Heterot.	73	3/91	(3.3)	0.9
Ao. ST.	29	2/41	(4.87)	0.8
Tricuspid At.	26	1/35	(2.85)	1.0
PPH	12	3/43	(6.97)	0.8
Truncus	21	2/16	(12.50)	0.7
MS, MI	15	1/21	(4.76)	0.8
Total	2962	67/3900		

VSD: ventricular septal defect; ASDII: auricular septal defect; TOF: tetralogy of Fallot; PDA: patent ductus arteriosus; PS: pulmonary stenosis; TGA: transposition of the great arteries; DORV; double outlet right ventricle; ECD; endocardial cushion defect; Dextro.; dextrocardia; Hoterot.; heterotaxy including asplenia and rudimentary spleen syndrome; APVD; anomalous pulmonary venous drainage; Ao. St.; aortic stenosis; Tricuspid At.; tricuspid atresia; PPH; primary pulmonary hypertension; MS; mitral stenosis; MI; mitral insufficiency.

expected recurrence risks. Observed values were remarkably increased compared to the incidence in the general population, and were distributed in the range of 1 to 5 percent, which is compatible with a multifactorial model. However, empiric risks were considerably lower than expected values at the top of the table, where the most common types of heart anomalies are shown. At the bottom of the table, where uncommon anomalies are listed, the observed values were considerably higher than expected recurrence risks. In theoretical recurrence risks and in Nora's study (1968), common lesions recur in first-degree relatives more commonly than uncommon lesions. Whether our finding is correct, or whether it is due to sampling bias, should be determined by a carefully planned family study using a larger sample.

Empiric risks in offspring of an affected individual were examined and are shown in Table 2. Because of the relatively small sample size, only ASDII gave a satisfactory value, which is very close to the expected recurrence risk.

These findings of familial incidence are hard to reconcile with single-gene dominant or recessive inheritance, but are compatible with a polygenic mode of inheritance.

Twin study. During the past 15 years, 113 pairs of twins have been examined, one or both of whom had common cardiac anomalies. Zygosity is based upon dermatoglyphic study and parents' statement. The rate of

TABLE 2. Observed and expected recurrence risks in offsprings. The calculation method is the same as that for Table 1.

Anomalies	Probands	Affected Offsprings		
		No.	(%)	Expected $\sqrt{p}$
VSD	60	0/75	—	4.9
ASDII	163	8/252	(3.17)	3.2
TOF	11	1/12	(8.33)	3.6
PDA	24	0/30	—	2.7
PS	13	0/15	—	1.5
ECD	6	1/6	(16.6)	1.3
Total	277	10/390	—	

TABLE 3. Twin study. Concordant rates of cardiac anomalies were examined in randomly ascertained twins with congenital heart disease. The concordance for monozygotic twins greatly exceeds the observed concordance for dizygotic twins, supporting the presence of genetic factors ($P<0.01$).

	Concordant CHD—CHD	Discordant CHD<Normal	Total
Our Data			
Monozygotic	11 (23.4%)	36	47
Dizygotic	3 (7.7%)	36	39
Unknown	2 (7.4%)	25	27
Total	16 (14.1%)	97	113
Nora's Data			
Monozygotic	6 (46.0%)	7	13
Dizygotic	1 (4.2%)	23	24

concordance for monozygotic twins is only 23.3 percent, while for dizygotic twins it is 7.69 percent ($P<0.01$) (Table 3). Of special importance is the fact that, given the same genetic background and similar intrauterine environment, more than 70 percent of identical twin sets are not concordant for the cardiac anomalies. The rate of concordance in fraternal twins is compatible to that of siblings born of separate pregnancies. These data provide evidence against a major gene or a major environmental teratogen in the etiology of common congenital heart disease.

Heritability. Using the method described by Falconer (1965), we calculated the heritability of several common cardiac lesions (Table 4). The method is based on an assumption of liability which expresses the combination of innate tendencies and external circumstances that make the person more or less likely to develop the disease in question. Whether an individual is affected or not depends on whether his liability exceeds or falls short of a fixed threshold. The correlation of liability between relatives leads to an estimate of the heritability of liability, which estimates the relative importance of hereditary factors as causes of differences in liability between individuals (Falconer, 1968).

Depending upon the type of cardiac anomaly, heritability was found in between 44 and 66 percent, averaging 57 percent (Table 4). Therefore the degree of genetic determination in common congenital heart disease may

TABLE 4. Heritability. General population incidence and relative frequency of each cardiac anomaly are estimated in the same way as in Table 1. A=observed number of affected individuals in siblings. N=total number of siblings. $Q=A/N$. b=regression coefficient of siblings on propositi. h=heritability of liability to the defects.

CHD	Proband	A	N	Q (%)	x	a	b	$h^2\pm$SE(%)
Gen. Popul.	—	—	—	0.21	2.863	3.156	—	
VSD	1241	18	1237	1.46	2.181	2.534	0.2161	43±6
Gen. Popul.	—	—	—	0.005	3.291	3.554	—	
ASDII	557	13	1110	1.17	2.283	2.627	0.2836	57±6
Gen. Popul.	—	—	—	0.045	3.353	3.613	—	
TOF	739	9	958	0.94	2.349	2.689	0.2779	56±7
Gen. Popul.	—	—	—	0.058	3.239	3.507	—	
PDA	295	8	408	1.96	2.081	2.445	0.3302	66±8
Gen. Popul.	—	—	—	0.06	3.239	3.507	—	
PS	123	3	199	1.51	2.167	2.522	0.3057	61±13
Gen. Popul.	—	—	—	0.255	2.807	3.104	—	
other CHD	571	22	746	2.95	1.869	2.281	0.3022	60±6

be estimated to be 57 percent; it may be greater, but it can never be less (Falconer, 1968). The remaining 43 percent would be the effects of environmental factors.

Genetic Factors

Thus, the multifactorial model with threshold can be reasonably well applied to the etiology of the major part of congenital heart disease among Japanese, as it has been to the disease among Caucasians by Nora (1968). However, as we have mentioned, the exact natures of genetic predispositions and of environmental teratogens are not well understood yet. In the future, studies on the etiology of congenital cardiac diseases should be aimed at clarifying these two factors.

Racial differences in the anatomic types of cardiac anomalies. Numerous clearcut genetic differences exist among racial groups. Racial differences in genetic predispositions could be expected to alter the incidence of some anomalies which are determined in a polygenic fashion. Racial comparisons of cardiovascular malformations may provide clues to the etiologic factors involved.

Available information regarding the overall incidence of cardiovascular anomalies does not appear to show critical racial differences among Caucasians (0.8–1.0 percent) (Mitchel, 1971; Hoffman, 1968), American Negroes (0.83 percent) (Mitchel, 1971), and Japanese (0.7 percent) (Neel, 1958). The incidence of particular cardiac anomalies was reported to show no significant difference between Negroes and Caucasians (Maron, 1973). Between Caucasians and Japanese, however, although no accurate information is available for a definitive comparison, clinical observations have led us to suspect that there might be racial differences in some particular types of cardiovascular anomalies, as shown in Figure 1 and Table 5. Possible sources of error in this type of comparison are several. A hospital-based study, like that shown in Figure 1, does not control the factors responsible for patients' choosing to come to the hospital. In a surveillance like that shown in Table 5 variations in available health care and in survey methods between nations or racial communities make racial comparisons difficult. Ideally, racial comparisons should be drawn from a well-designed prospective survey among representatives of different races in the same country as well as those in different countries.

Another important point to be considered in a study on etiology is that

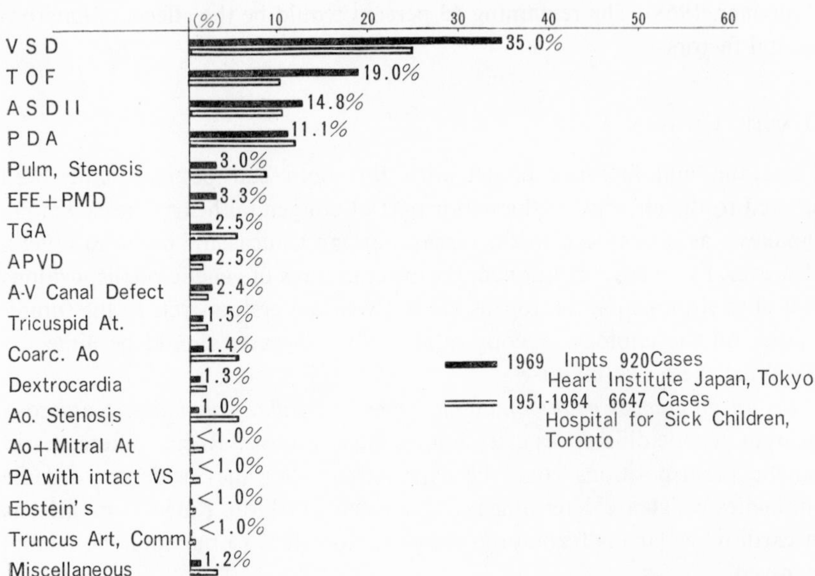

FIG. 1. Relative incidence of cardiac anomalies in cardiac clinics. Racial comparison was based on the relative frequency of each cardiac anomaly at hospitals with facilities for cardiovascular treatment.

TABLE 5. Relative incidence of cardiac anomalies at school age. Relative frequency of individual cardiac anomalies was determined in 1,262 patients who were found in a survey of 533,829 Japanese school children aged 6 to 12 years (Ando 1975b). It was compared to that of 291 patients who were found in a survey of 130,936 school children in Liverpool, England (Hay 1966).

	Japan %	Liverpool %
VSD	44.0	28.1
ASD	22.0	15.1
PDA	11.6	14.1
PS	5.7	17.5
TOF	5.6	3.8
AS	—	11.7
COARC.	—	2.5
OTHER CHD's	10.7	7.2

the individual diagnostic entity should be genetically and embryologically pure. However, the classification of congenital heart disease in use at present is mainly based on clinical similarity. Therefore, many diagnostic entities may include embryologically and anatomically heterogeneous groups. Racial comparisons should be performed within the anatomic types of each diagnostic entity. To our knowledge, studies on racial differences have never been performed within the anatomic types of specific categories of cardiac malformations.

Isolated ventricular septal defect. Anatomic types of simple ventricular septal defect (VSD), unassociated with tetralogy of Fallot (TOF), transposition of great arteries (TGA), or other complex cardiac anomalies (except coarctation, interruption, PDA, and ASDII), were analyzed in 146 Japanese specimens. These specimens are part of the collection of the Heart Institute of Japan, which includes 1,500 specimens with congenital heart disease. The data were compared with two autopsy series on Caucasians: the one is reported by Goor *et al.* (1970), and the other is a series examined by one of the authors (MA) at Children's Hospital Medical Center, Boston (1975a).

The classification of the anatomic types is according to the location of the defect (Figures 2, 3). There are three developmental components in the ventricular septum: infundibular, membranous, and muscular sinus septum. The muscular sinus septum is divided into an inflow smooth septum and an apical trabeculated septum (Goor, 1973). VSD can occur in each septal component and also at the junction of each septal component. The cases of the former type are simple punch-out VSD due to defective development of the septal component. The same mechanism is also present in the latter;

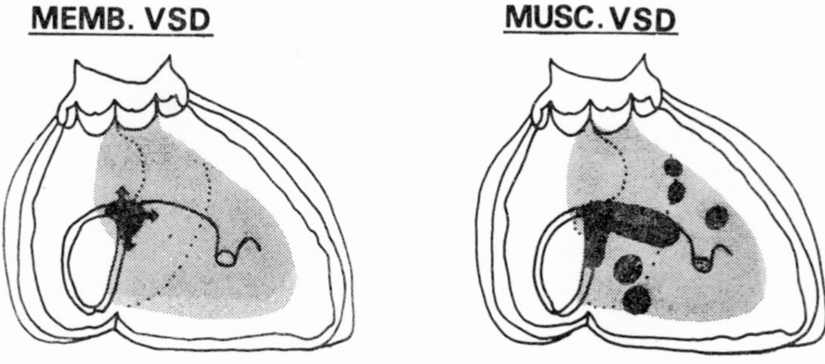

FIG. 2. Membranous and muscular VSD

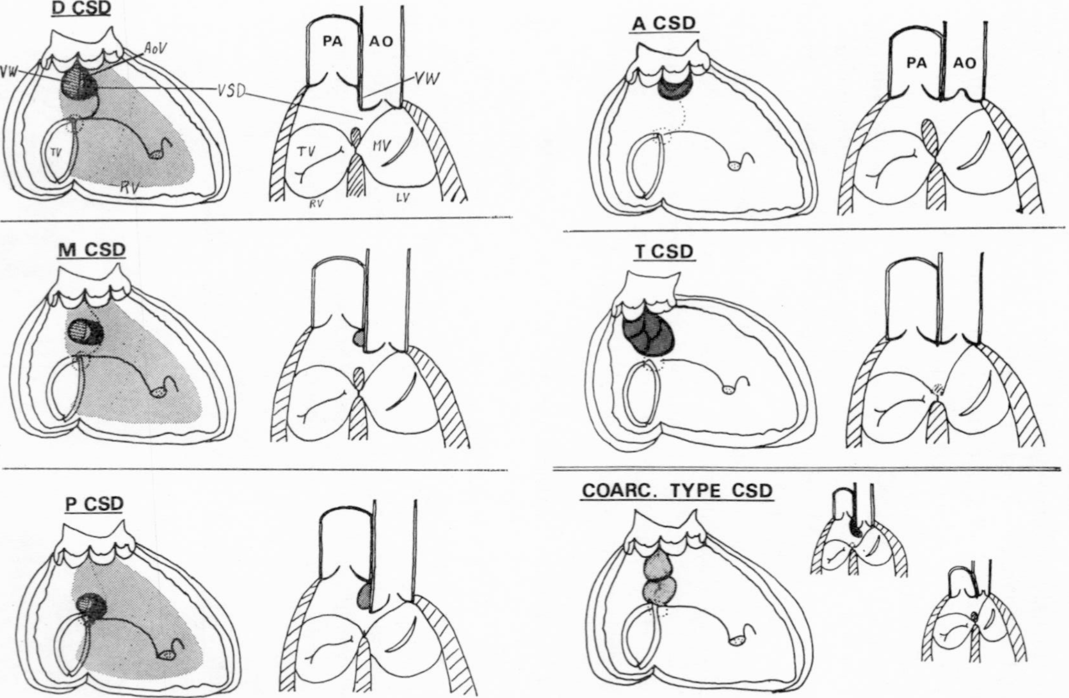

FIG. 3. Anatomic types of infundibular VSD. Right ventricular views are shown on the right side of each panel. On the left side, the schematic presentations of frontal cut surface perpendicular to each septal component are shown. CSD is an abbreviation of conus septum defect. D, M, P, A, and T are distal, mid-, proximal, anterior, and total, respectively. Coarc.=Coarctation of aorta. VW=Wall of sinus Valsalva. AoV=Aortic valve. TV=Tricuspid valve. MV=Mitral valve. RV=right ventricle. LV=left ventricle.

however, significant cases of the latter type are due to malalignment of the adjacent septa, usually inolving cono-ventricular or cono-truncal alignment, which is the most vital part of the cardiac anomalies.

Infundibular VSD has five subtypes. The first three are distal, mid-, and proximal conus septum defects, which are generally simple punch-out VSD and are frequently associated with aortic regurgitation due to prolapsed aortic cusp into VSD. The last two subtypes are anterior and total conus septum defects, which are usually due to malalignment of the relating septa. Membranous and muscular VSD are simple punchout VSD in those septa or fusion lines. Figures 2 and 3 show the schema of each type.

As shown in Table 6, infundibular VSD is almost twice as frequent in

TABLE 6. Racial comparison in relative frequencies of antomic type of simple VSD.

	Japanese *1 146 VSD's in 145 Specimens Percent (No of cases)		American *2 112 VSD's in 101 Specimens Precent (No of cases)		American *3 157 VSD's in 150 Specimens Percent (No of cases)	
Infundibular VSD	**59.6** (87)		**27.7** (31)		**31.8** (50)	
Anterior conus septum defect (Genuine Supra-cristal VSD)		2.1 (3)		0		4.5 (7)
Distal conus septum defect		**23.3** (34)		**1.8** (2)		**1.3** (2)
Mid-conus septum defect		2.1 (3)		4.5 (5)		3.2 (5)
Proximal conus septum defect		28.7 (42)		19.6 (22)		21.5 (34)
Total conus spetum defect		3.4 (5)		1.8 (2)		1.3 (2)
Membranous canal type VSD	24.7 (36)		19.6 (22)		28.7 (45)	
Atrio-ventricular VSD		0		1.8 (2)		0
Membranous VSD		23.3 (34)		16.9 (19)		28.0 (44)
Canal VSD		1.4 (2)		0.9 (1)		0.7 (1)
Muscular VSD	**15.7** (23)		**52.7** (59)		**39.5** (62)	
RV inflow VSD (smooth VSD)		14.3 (21)		49.1 (55)		33.8 (53)
Apical VSD (trabeculated VSD)		1.4 (2)		3.6 (4)		5.7 (9)

*1. Japanese series. *2. From literature (Goor, 1973).
*3. Caucasian series at Children's Hospital, Boston.

Japanese specimens as in Caucasian specimens; distal conus septum defect, which is most often associated with prolapsing aortic insufficiency, is especially frequent. In contrast, muscular VSD is commoner in Caucasian specimens. Excess infundibular VSD in Japanese corresponds well to the high incidence of aortic valves dislocating into VSD and aortic regurgitation, which is one of the most important clinical problems in Japanese with cardiac anomalies.

Coarctation or interruption-type VSD. Several types of VSD are significantly associated with coarctation or interruption of aorta. Common anatomic features of this type of VSD are posterior deviation of conus septum or truncal septum due to malalignment, which induces subaortic narrowing due to deviated conus or truncal septum, aortic levoposition, and VSD. Therefore, during fetal life, aortic flow may decrease and hypoplasia of the aortic isthmus may result. The four subtypes of the defect are shown in Figure 4. Figure 5 gives examples of some subtypes.

Subpulmonary VSD of the coarctation-interruption type is remarkably frequent among Japanese (47 percent); in Caucasians it is only 9 percent. Subcristal VSD of the coarctation-interruption type is twice as frequent in Caucasian specimens as in Japanese specimens (Table 7).

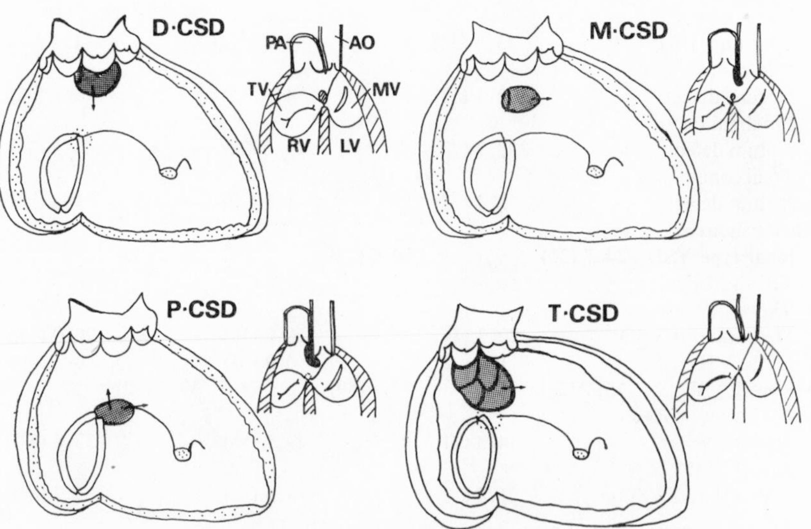

FIG. 4. Schema of anatomic types of coarctation-interruption type VSD.

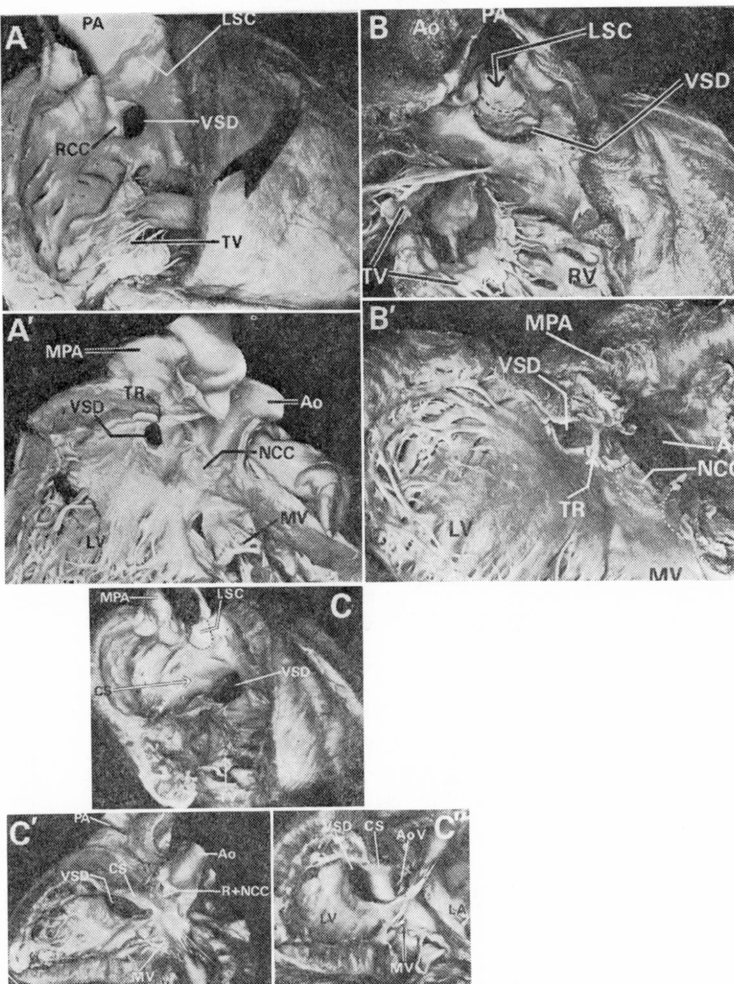

FIG. 5. Examples of coarctation-interruption-type VSD. A: Distal CSD with posterior deviation of truncal septum (TR). B: Distal CSD with anterior extension. C: Proximal CSD with posterior deviation of conus septum (CS). A′, B′, and C′: The left ventricular view of each case, as shown in these panels, demonstrates that the truncal septum (A′, B′) or conal septum (C′) is on the left ventricle due to posterior deviation of the septum very close to the mitral valve (MV). In C″, when the left ventricular outflow tract is viewed from the cardiac apex, the subaortic region and aortic valve (AoV) is remarkably narrowed behind the deviated crista (CS), and in front of the crista, large VSD leads into the right ventricular outflow tract. All cases had coarctation of aorta. LSC=left septal cusp of pulmonary valve. RCC=right coronary cusp. MPA=main pulmonary artery. NCC=noncoronary cusp. LA=left atrium.

TABLE 7. Frequency of anatomic types of coarctation-interruption-type VSD. Japanese series is from the collection of CHD specimens in our hospital. Caucasian series is from the Children's Hospital, Boston. All cases had isthmic hypoplasia, coarctation of aorta, or interruption of aorta (Int).

	Japanese			White		
	No.	(%)		No.	(%)	
D. CSD	17	(47)	(Int: 1)	3	(9)	
M. CSD	2	(6)		2	(6)	(Int: 2)
P. CSD	16	(44)	(Int: 4)	26	(82)	(Int: 11)
T. CSD	1	(3)		1	(3)	
Total No.	36			32		

TABLE 8. Tetralogy of Fallot and subpulmonary VSD with pulmonary stenosis. Racial comparisons were performed in surgical series and autopsy series between Japanese and Caucasians. Clinical tetralogy includes both morphological TOF and CSD+PS.

	Japanese	White (American)
I. Surgical Series		
Clinical Tetralogy	312 cases (1971–1973)*	Classical TOF Morphology
Subpulmonary VSD with PS	30 cases (9.6%)	very rare
II. Autopsy Series		
Clinical Tetralogy	131 cases (in 1050 specimens)**	111 cases (in 1500 specimens)***
Subpulmonary VSD with PS	22 cases (16.8%)	2 cases (1.8%)

* Surgical cases at the Heart Institute of Japan, 1971 to 1973.
** Autopsy series at the Heart Institute.
*** Autopsy series at Children's Hospital, Boston.

Tetralogy of Fallot and Subpulmonary VSD with pulmonary stenosis. In Japanese patients with clinical signs and symptoms of tetralogy of Fallot (TOF), there are two different anatomic types; one is morphologically classical TOF, and the other is subpulmonary VSD with pulmonary stenosis (CSD+PS), in which the conus septum is totally or subtotally absent and the truncal septum deviates anteriorly, inducing pulmonary valve ring stenosis. CSD+PS is not rare in Japanese patients with clinical signs of TOF (Table 8). However, this type of case appears to be paticularly uncommon in Caucasians (Satyanarayana, 1974; Ando, 1974).

These data suggest that the racial differences may be present in the anatomic types of several diagnostic entities of cardiac anomalies. The direct implication of this hypothesis is twofold: (1) Racial differences in genetic predispositions for abnormal cardiac morphogenesis seem to exist between Caucasians and Japanese. (2) Etiologic heterogeneity appears to be present in some of the clinical diagnostic entities of cardiac anomalies, as previously shown in VSD and TOF. Therefore, for the purpose of etiologic study, anatomic types of each diagnostic group should be reconsidered. For example, VSD should be subdivided according to the location and presence or absence of septal malalignment, probably into at least three major types—Eisenmenger VSD, coarctation or interruption-type VSD, and simple punchout VSD—each of which includes several subtypes according to location. In TOF, there are two types, classical TOF and CSD+PS. Each of these anatomic types can be diagnosed by careful clinical observation and angiography.

Cono-truncal malformation with peculiar facial appearance. In our cardi-

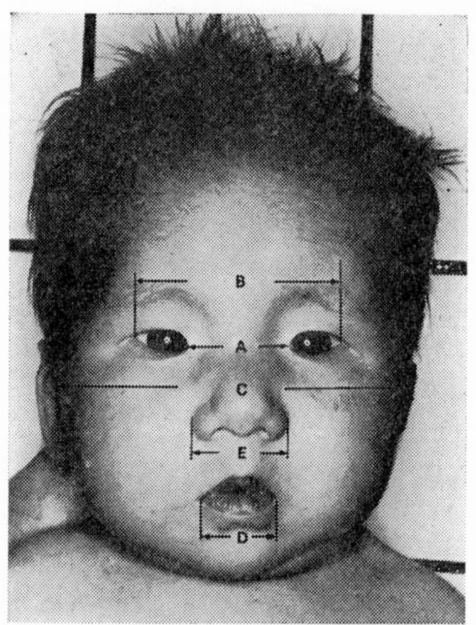

A: Inner canthal distance
B: Outer canthal distance
C: Facial transverse width
D: Oral width
E: Nasal width

FIG. 6. Cono-truncal faces. Peculiar facial features are not rarely associated with TOF in Japanese. Several anthropometrical analyses were done to demonstrate ocular hypertelorism (A/C), small eye fissures (B–A/C), small mouth (D/E, D/C), etc., and compared with those of normal children of comparable age groups. Significant differences were observed in all of these calculations.

TABLE 9. Characteristic features of cono-trauncal faces. Hypertelorism with bloated upper eyelids and small eye fissures, low nose root, small mouth (sometimes smaller than nasal width) and high arched palate, nasal voice, and deformed ear lobes are characteristic of cono-truncal faces. Short stature and mild mental retardation are occassionally seen.

Ocular Hypertlorism	100%
Narrow Eye Fissures	100%
Low Nose Root	100%
Small Mouth	97%
Bloated Eyelids	93%
Nasal Voice	100%
High Arched Palate	70%
Strabismus Convergence	11%
Deformed Ear Lobes	73%

ovascular clinics, patients with TOF were occasionally observed in association with peculiar facial features, as shown in Figure 6. Facial measurements as indicated in Figure 6 were performed in 30 cases of this association, and compared to those of 120 normal children of similar sex and age distribution (Kinouchi, 1976). The facial features were highly specific for the pateints with TOF, and can be called cono-truncal faces (Table 9). Small stature and mental ratardation are occasionally seen. Some of the parents and siblings of the patients with cono-truncal faces showed several features of these faces, but without cardiac involvements. Therefore, the patients with the faces may have inherited a higher liability to cono-truncal malformations. Study of families with this association promises some clues about the etiology of the defects.

Dermatoglyphic Analyses. Fingerprint patterns, axial triradius, simian lines, and hallucal patterns of the soles were examined in 522 patients with common CHD, and in some of their parents (Ando, 1972, 1973). These were compared with those of normal Japanese. Statistically significant differences were observed between these groups ($P < 0.05$). In fingerprints, the ulnar loop (U) was consistently the most frequent pattern in CHD group, while in the normals, the whorl (W) was the commonest pattern (CHD: W 43.5 percent, U 50.5 percent; control: W 48.7 percent, U 46.5 percent). The incidence of high axial triradius (t′ or t″) was significantly increased among CHD patients (CHD 48.9 percent, control 40.2 percent). Frequencies of simian and semi-simian lines increased in CHD group (CHD 39.8 percent, control 21.5 percent). In hallucal patterns, tibial arches and distal loops with ridge counts less than 20 were more frequently observed among CHD patients than among normal controls (CHD 35.8 percent, control 21.1 percent).

These slight but consistent differences were similarly observed in the parents of the patients with CHD. Therefore, some of the patients with CHD may have inherited a higher liability to abnormal dermatoglyphics from their parents. Conversely, those patients whose dermatoglyphics are unlike those of their parents might have had more environmental teratogenic insults during the critical developmental period of hands and soles, which, in part, might well have overlapped into cardiovascular development. Quantitative genetic studies of dermatoglyphics are necessary in order to separate these two extreme groups: CHD patients with higher liability to genetic factors and those having been exposed to environmental teratogens for abnormal dermatoglyphics.

Environmental Factors

Maternal histories of abnormal episodes during the first trimester of pregnancy were retrospectively examined for 272 Japanese patients with established diagnoses of cardiac anomalies. The results were compared with those of 204 babies who were born during April 1972 and February 1973 at the Gynecologic Clinic of St. Luke's International Hospital, Tokyo. All controls were Japanese without cardiac anomalies. Differences between the two groups were significant ($P<0.01$) with respect to the presence or absence of threatened abortion other abnormal maternal conditions which include various conditions not indicated in figures.

To confirm these findings, another study is in progress. In this study, normal siblings of the index cases were used as a control series. An interim calculation reveals significant differences as to the presence or absence of maternal episodes (Fig. 7), including infectious diseases, anemia, other maternal conditions, treatment with antibiotics and sedatives during the first trimester. Significant difference was not revealed as to hormone therapy and threatened abortion ($P<0.05$). As these studies are retrospective and preliminary and the control series are not completely satisfactory, it is hard to reach any conclusions from the above preliminary analysis. However, these data strongly suggest the need for further studies, preferably in a prospective form concerning abnormal episodes during the first trimester, in order to demonstrate environmental teratogens which are relevant to the etiology of cardiac malformations.

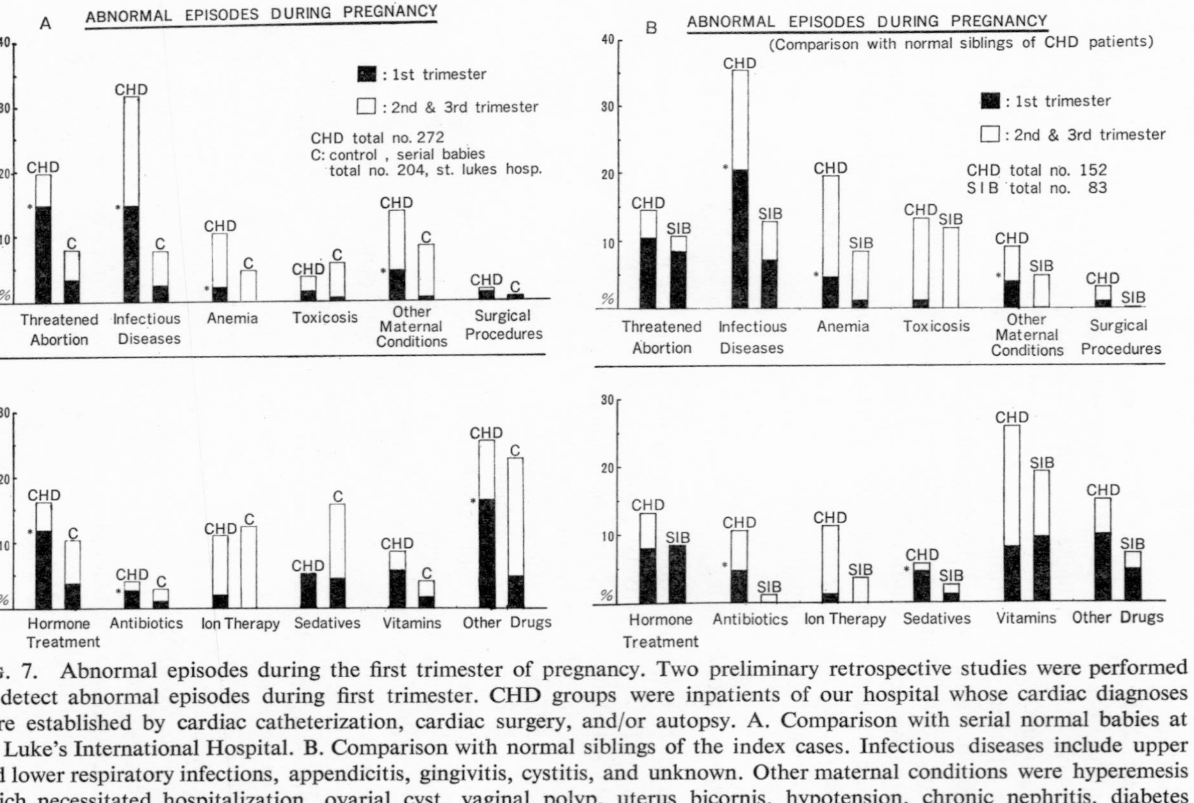

FIG. 7. Abnormal episodes during the first trimester of pregnancy. Two preliminary retrospective studies were performed to detect abnormal episodes during first trimester. CHD groups were inpatients of our hospital whose cardiac diagnoses were established by cardiac catheterization, cardiac surgery, and/or autopsy. A. Comparison with serial normal babies at St. Luke's International Hospital. B. Comparison with normal siblings of the index cases. Infectious diseases include upper and lower respiratory infections, appendicitis, gingivitis, cystitis, and unknown. Other maternal conditions were hyperemesis which necessitated hospitalization, ovarial cyst, vaginal polyp, uterus bicornis, hypotension, chronic nephritis, diabetes mellitus, valvular heart disease, and chronic diarrhea. Other drugs were calcium compounds, salicylates, and unknown. These were observed in CHD groups during the first trimester.

Summary

There is a growing body of indirect evidence showing that multifactorial inheritance with threshold is a plausible genetic model of many common malformations. A major group of congenital heart disease also appears to conform to the multifactorial model. To demonstrate the exact nature of genetic predispositions which may predominantly relate to the abnormal morphogenesis as well as of environmental factors which may lower the threshold for a particular defect in morphogenesis, several studies were undertaken at our Heart Institute, and some of the preliminary results of these studies have been presented.

Possible etiologic heterogeneity was shown in the categories of VSD and TOF by racial comparisons of the anatomic types of each category. To isolate the genetic as well as environmental factors, the classification of cardiac anomalies for etiologic studies should be reconsidered according to the morphological and embryological bases of the defects. Some evidence was obtained as to the genetic predispositions, by inter-racial comparisons of anatomic types of each cardiac anomaly, and by family studies of such abnormal stigmata as cono-truncal faces and dermatoglyphic features.

At the same time it is felt that systematic observations of abnormal episodes during early pregnancy should be carried out in order to demonstrate multiple and subtle environmental factors responsible for the etiology.

Acknowledgments

We wish to thank Dr. R. Van Praagh for giving us permission to examinine heart specimens in the cardiac registry, CHMC, Boston, and Dr. T. Yamamoto and Dr. E. Suzuki for their cooperation in the study of abnormal episodes in early pregnancy.

REFERENCES

Ando, M., Mori, K., and Takao, A. 1969. Study on familial occurrence of congenital heart disease. *Jap. Heart J.* **33**: 967.

Ando, M. 1972. Dermatoglyphics in congenital heart disease. *Jap. J. Hum. Genet.* **18**: 73.

Ando, M. 1973. Genetic and environmental interaction for the genesis of congenital heart disease: Study on empiric recurrence risks and dermatoglyphics. *Cong. Anom.* **13**: 147.

Ando, M. 1974. Subpulmonary ventricular septal defect with pulmonary stenosis. *Circulation* **50**: 412.

Ando, M., and Takao, A. 1975a. Anatomic variabilities between races in some major cardiac anomalies. *Teratology* **12**: 194.

Ando, M. 1975b. Epidemiology of congenital heart disease, in *Rinsho-Junkanki-Koza*, vol. 2, p. 83. Kanehara, Tokyo, Japan.

Falconer, D. S. 1960. *Introduction to quantative genetics.* Boyd, Edinburgh, Scotland.

Falconer, D. S. 1965. The inheritance of liability to certain diseases, estimated from the incidence among relatives. *Ann. Hum. Genet.* (London) **29**: 51.

Goor, D. A., Lillehei, C. W., Rees, R., and Edwards, J. E. 1970. Isolated ventricular septal defect. Developmental basis for various types and presentations of classification. *Chest* **58**: 468.

Hay, J. D. 1966. Population and clinic studies of congenital heart disease in Liverpool. *Br. Med. J.* **2**: 661.

Hoffman, J. I. E. 1968. Natural history of congenital heart disease, problems in its assessment with special reference to ventricular septal defects. *Circulation* **37**: 97.

Kinouchi, A., Mori, K., Ando, M., and Takao, A. 1976. Facial appearance of patients with cono-truncal anomalies. *Pediatrics of Japan* **17**: 84.

Maron, B. J., Applefeld, J. M., and Krovetz, L. J. 1973. Racial frequencies in congenital heart disease. *Circulation* **47**: 359.

Mitchel, S. C., Korones, S. B., and Brendes, H. W. 1971. Congenital heart disease in 56,109 births: Incidence and natural history. *Circulation* **43**: 97.

Mori, K., Ando, M., and Takao, A. 1973. Genetic aspects of congenital heart disease. *Jap. Heart J.* **36**: 90.

Neel, J. V. 1958. A study of major congenital defects in Japanese infants. *Amer. J. Hum. Genet.* **10**: 398.

Nora, J. J. 1968. Maltifactorial inheritance hypothesis for the etiology of congenital heart diseases: The genetic-environment interaction. *Circulation* **38**: 604.

Satyanarayana Rao, B. M., and Edwards, J. E. 1974. Conditions simulating the tetralogy of Fallot. *Circulation* **49**: 173.

DISCUSSION 1

Programmed Cell Death in Bulbar Cushion of Developing Heart

Naomasa Okamoto

Since Ernst in 1926 published the first comprehensive study on the occurrence of cell death during the embryogenesis of various organs in various locations, many authors have emphasized the importance or utility of physiological cell death during embryonic development.

Concerning cell death in developing cardiovascular systems, Pexieder has systematically studied cell death in the morphogenesis of the chick embryonic heart and made a list of cell death zones appearing during cardiac development. It has been suggested that all cell death caused by exogenous agents during the development of the cardiovascular system may play some kind of a role in its abnormal formation, but the relationship between cell death and the type of cardiovascular anomalies which were eventually formed has not yet been clarified. The main object of the present report is to clarify the role of the physiological cell death in the conus during the formation of embryonic rat hearts in their normal and abnormal conditions, from both genetic and environmental points of view.

Material and Methods

Rats of the Donryu strain were used. Males and females were kept in a cage overnight, and the 0 day of gestation was determined by finding sperm in the vaginal smears on the following morning. Pregnant rats were exposed to a single dose of 130 rads of whole-body neutron radiation 8 days after conception.

Figure 1 shows the morphological changes of conus ridges in the control group.

On the 12th day the sinistral and dextral conus ridges are clearly seen to develop. On the 13th day the fusion of the conus ridge is not yet seen. The sinistroventral conus ridge (black shading) is always related to the anterior margin of the bulboventricular foramen, whereas the dextrodorsal

Department of Geneticopathology, Research Institute for Nuclear Medicine and Biology, Hiroshima, Japan.

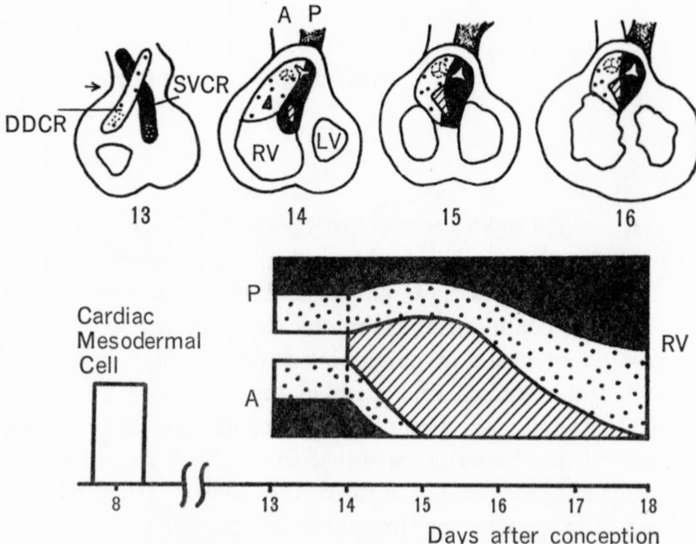

FIG. 1. Top—semidiagrammatic illustrations of the conus ridges in the control group. Arrow is truncobulbar curvature.
Bottom—diagrammatic illustrations of the absorption of the subaortic conus ridge. ——; sinistroventral conus ridge, ——; dextrodorsal conus ridge, A; aorta, P; pulmonary artery, RV; right ventrical and LV; left ventricle.

conus ridge (stippled) is always related to the right of the bulboauriculo-ventricular ledge. Both ridges are twisted together at the level of "truncobular curvature" (→).

On the 14th day, the septation of aorta and pulmonary artery becomes conspicuous; the conus is also shortened with further development, and the primordia of aortic valves are located at the dorsal part of the fused conus ridge under the primordia of pulmonary valves.

The lower part of Figure 1 illustrates the schematic drawing of changes in the developing bulbar ridge. The hatched portions show the cell death focus. P is the portion of primordium of the pulmonary valve. A is the portion of primordium of the aortic valve.

RV is the right ventricle. The cell death which begins to appear from the latter half of the 13th day of gestation forms foci at the 14th day which gradually increase in size, becoming very dense from the 15th to the 16th day. They decrease rapidly on the 17th day, disappearing completely on the 18th day. These cell-deaths are found in the proximal inferior subaortic conus ridges. The cell death focus is seen extending from the primordium of the aortic valves to the fused area of the conus ridge under the primordium of the pulmonary valves and toward the proximal part of the aorticipulmonary septum. This focus disappears at the stage in which the aortic valve is connected with the left atrioventricular endocardial cushions. Therefore, the aorta is seen to migrate gradually above the left ventricle as the cell-death foci decrease. These data suggest that the occurrence of cell death in the conus is related to the migration of the aorta into the left ventricle.

It is reasonable to assume that cell-death masses in the conus ridge occur not by chance, but by a genetically controlled program, because the site where cell death occurs in the normal process of cardiac development is found at the fixed loci. Furthermore, the extent of death regions is constant. The cell-death masses in the conus ridge appear and disappear in the same place and at the same stage of development.

The lower part of Figure 2 shows the schematic drawing of a normal case

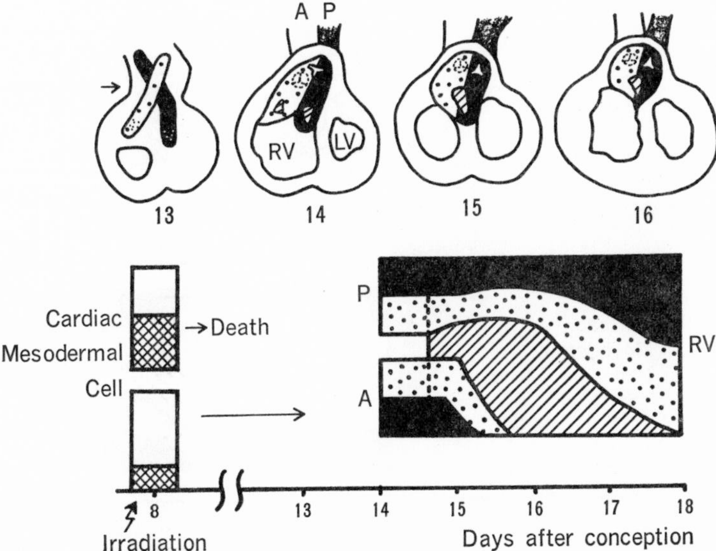

FIG. 2. Semidiagrammatic (top) and diagrammatic (bottom) illustrations of the conus ridges of normal cases in irradiated group.
——; direct cell death caused by irradiation.

in the irradiated group. The appearance of cell death masses in the conus ridge is perhaps controlled. Compared with those in control groups, cell deaths in the experimental group occur about 24 hours later; the size and number of cell death foci are smaller compared to those of controls, but the time of disappearance of cell death is the same in both the control and experimental groups.

Figure 3 shows the changes of cell death focus in the double outlet right ventricle (DORV). In the control group on the 15th day, cell death is observed in the conus ridge at the aortic side, but in DORV cases, the inferior conus ridge under the aortic valve is on the right side of the pulmonary valve, and the cell-death mass extends from the developing aorticopulmonary septum to the proximal part of the inferior conus ridge under the pulmonary valve. This indicates that subaortic conus ridges may remain at their original foci, thereby producing a disturbance of aortic migration into the left ventricle.

Figure 4 shows the changes of cell-death focus in complete transposition of the aorta. The cell-death foci are found in the subpulmonary conus ridge

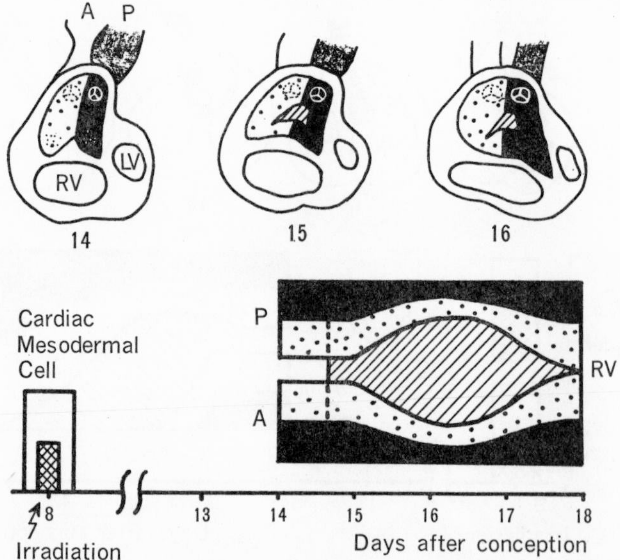

FIG. 3. Semidiagrammatic (top) and diagrammatic (bottom) illustrations of the cell death focus of conus ridges in the case of double outlet right ventricle.

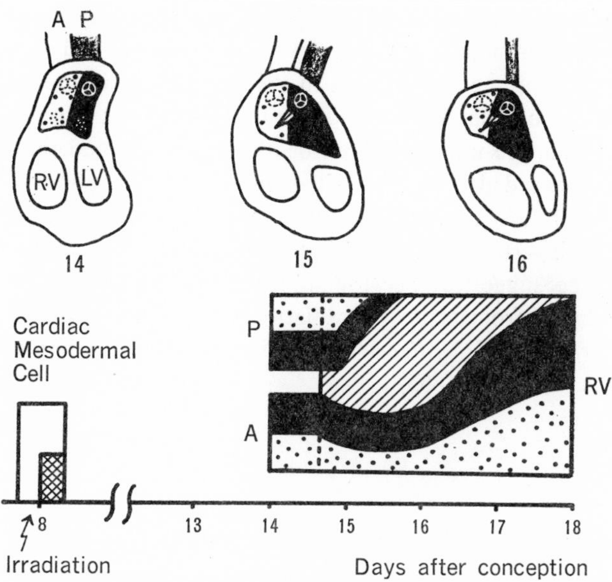

FIG. 4. Semidiagrammatic (top) and diagrammatic (bottom) illustrations of the cell-death focus of the conus ridges in the case of complete transposition of the great arteries.

situated inferiorly and dorsally to the left side of the aortic valve. No cell death foci are found in the subaortic distal bulbar ridge in this anomaly. This shows that the pulmonary artery may migrate into the left ventricle.

Therefore, definite patterns of cell death in cardiovascular anomalies occur in different places and to a different extent in comparison with normal cases. These facts provide us with grounds for considering the cell death which occurs in a definite type of cardiovascular anomaly as a kind of genetically programmed phenomenon caused by neutron.

Neutron is irradiated at the period of the development of cardiac mesodermal cells in our experiment. The cell death caused by direct irradiation in this stage is different from that which is taken up in the present report. The direct cell death disappears after 24 hours and the damages caused by irradiation may be repaired. After this period, normal or abnormal heart develops and conus ridges are formed. Some cell deaths begin to appear in the conus ridges and gradually increase with age. Morphology of this type of cell death is different from the direct cell death seen shortly after irradiation.

As mentioned above, differences in programmed cell death between normal and experimental groups may be the amount and site of the cell death: the programmed cell deaths in the conus ridge in the experimental group appeared one day later than those in controls, but disappeared at the same time; also, the number of cell deaths was small, and the position of the cell deaths tended to have a mirror image to the controls.

At present the reason for these phenomena is not known, but the possibility of a inverted change of induction potentiality to form normal hearts may be suggested, because of the decrease in number of cardiac mesodermal cells from neutron-irradiation. (See *Developmental and Physiological Correlates of Cardiac Muscle*, edited by M. Lieberman and T. Sano. Raven Press, 1975, p. 51–65)

DISCUSSION 2

Effects of Radiation on Genetically Programmed Development of the Heart

Takayoshi Ikeda

In relation to Dr. Ando's paper concerning congenital heart diseases, the influences of environmental factors on the genetically programmed developmental process were discussed.

Genetically determined developmental process in the normal heart may be affected completely or partially, and permanently or temporarily, by some environmental factors during the organogenetic period. Methodologically, a disturbance of normal genetic program could be demonstrated by isoenzyme analysis, such as lactate dehydrogenase (LDH) isoenzyme, which is a suitable indicator of embryonic developmental process.

In radiation-induced cardiovascular anomalies of the rat, LDH isoenzyme pattern of the heart tissue and whole body extracts was temporarily affected shortly after irradiation. However, the recovery of isoenzyme pattern was observed uhtil 6 days after irradiation, and no abnormal patterns were seen thereafter, although the lower activity of the enzyme which might be caused by cell death following irradiation was noted. On the other hand, some cases may have retained permanently the variant type of LDH isoenzyme.

These findings indicate that temporal or permanent effects of normal gene expression in developmental process and target cell damage by environmental factors such as radiation may be involved in the mechanisms of teratogenesis.

Nagasaki University School of Medicine, Nagasaki, Japan.

Factors Influencing the Occurrence of Cleft Lip and Cleft Palate*

F. C. Fraser

For some years we have been studying cleft palate and cleft lip, induced experimentally in mice, as a model for the analysis of gene-environment interactions. Cleft palate has been shown to be a multifactorial, threshold character, and a number of the factors involved have been identified (Fraser, 1969).

Figure 1 is a diagrammatic and oversimple representation of the concept (Fraser, 1976). In order to fuse successfully, the palate shelves must move from their vertical positions on either side of the tongue to a horizontal position above the tongue, and then extend toward the midline until they meet. If they do not achieve the horizontal before a certain critical stage of development, they are unable to meet, or unable to fuse when they do meet, and cleft palate will result. This critical stage, therefore, represents a threshold. In a given population of mouse embryos, the stage of shelf movement can be considered a continuously distributed variable, and the threshold separates those embryos in which the horizontal is reached in time, and whose palates will be normal, from those in which it occurs too late, and whose palates will be cleft. The position of an embryo in the distribution relative to the threshold determines its suceptibility to cleft lip. For example, the A/J inbred mouse strain is relatively susceptible to the production of cleft palate by cortisone and 6-aminonicotinamide, and palate closure occurs at a later stage than it does in the comparatively resistant C57BL/6 strain. In a series of crosses, there was good correspondence between initiation of palate closure and resistance to cortisone (Trasler, 1965).

Department of Biology and Pediatrics, McGill University, and the Medical Research Council Medical Genetics Group, The Montreal Children's Hospital, Montreal, Canada.

* Publication No. 446 from the McGill University-Montreal Children's Hospital Research Institute.

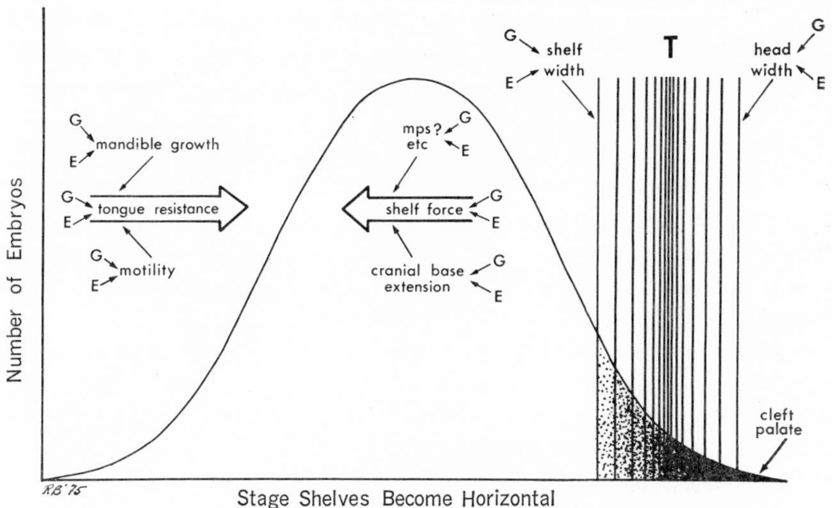

FIG. 1. Diagram illustrating the multifactorial/threshold concept for cleft palate. The interaction between shelf force and tongue resistance determines the stage in development at which the shelves move to the horizontal. The threshold is the latest stage at which fusion can occur, and beyond which cleft palate will result. Shelf force, tongue resistance, and position of threshold are all influenced by genetic and environmental variation.

There is an intrinsic shelf force which progressively builds up in the shelves so that they (normally) overcome the resistance of the intervening tongue and move to the horizontal. The stage at which they do this is determined by the relative strengths of shelf force and tongue resistance.

The exact nature of the shelf force is still not known, though there are various hypotheses to choose from (Burdi *et al.*, 1972; Verrusio, 1972; Long *et al.*, 1973; Zimmerman *et al.*, 1975), but there are numerous factors that can alter it, both genetic and environmental. Tongue resistance is also influenced by many things, including its motility, mechanical pressure (as in oligohydramnios), interference with its forward movement (as in cleft lip embryos, or as a result of micrognathia, or an unusually short snout), and both genetic and environmental factors can act on each of these. The position of the threshold is also variable, depending on the width of the shelves and the width of the head, and these are also presumably influenced by both genetic and environmental factors. Other elements in this multifactorial system no doubt remain to be identified. One intriguing discovery is the association of the H-2 locus with susceptibility to cortisone-induced cleft palate in the mouse (Bonner and Slavkin, 1975); it will be interesting to see whether histocompatibility differences are significant in human facial clefts and other malformations (Erickson, 1975).

For cleft lip the situation is not so clear, but a hypothesis has been developed relating certain factors in embryonic face shape to susceptibility (Trasler, 1968). It is suggested that successful formation of the primary palate depends on the maintenance of the contiguity between the medial and lateral nasal processes during the formation of the nasal fin and the fusion of their epithelia at the lower end of the nasal pit. In the (susceptible) A/Jax mouse, the medial nasal processes are more medially placed than in the (resistant) C57BL/6 mouse (Trasler and Leong, 1976), suggesting that because of the greater distance from the lateral processes the required degree of contiguity is not maintained, epithelial fusion is not complete, and the bridge between the two processes breaks down, leading to cleft lip. In mice heterozygous for the "dancer" gene, which are also susceptible to cleft lip, the medial process is unusually small, leading to the same result. In embryos in which cleft lip is produced by treatment with 6-aminonicotinamide on day 10½, the lateral process is reduced in thickness. So, as in the cases of cleft palate, it appears that the defect can be produced by many mechanisms or (and this is probably the most common situation) by a combination of several different mechanisms, interacting to produce the threshold effect.

In man, in spite of much effort and many claims, relatively few specific environmental factors have been identified. The situation is well reviewed by Saxen (1975a, b), who has also provided some instructive data. Information (only partly retrospective) gathered by the Finnish Register of Congenital Malformations on 791 women who had given birth to children with cleft lip and/or palate was compared to that for matched controls in two consecutive samples. Statistically significant effects of paternal age, socioeconomic class, season of birth, previous maternal pelvic X-ray, and psychological stress during pregnancy seen in the first sample disappeared in the second sample. This emphasizes that, particularly when a large number of comparisons are made, some "statistically significant" differences may be random fluctuations, with no biological significance. It also leaves us wondering which result was the correct one. Reports of parental age effects have been conflicting (Perry and Fraser, 1972), and these effects appear to occur mainly, if not entirely, when the clefts are associated with other malformations (Hay, 1967), suggesting that they may reflect an admixture of chromosomal syndromes and dominant mutations.

The most interesting associations in the Finnish study were with influenza, fever, and the intake of certain drugs (salicylates, other antipyretics, opiates, penicillins, antihistamines, and antianxiety drugs). Maternal memory bias was probably not an important factor, as the associations occurred only in the first trimester, and some drugs (e.g., cyclizines) did not show the association. Statistical analysis of the associations between these factors showed that the association of fever with clefts could be accounted for by its association with influenza and salicylates. However, the association of influenza with clefts (previously noted in several other studies) could not be accounted for by its association with salicylates, or vice versa. Each had an independent effect. The situation is complex, and other studies of this type are needed.

A correlation of cleft lip with influenza epidemics was shown by Leck (1971), but only in epidemics due to recurrences of familiar viral strains. Moreover, there was no relation to a particular stage of gestation, suggesting that the epidemic was influencing the survival of embryos with cleft lip rather than causing cleft lip. A preferential survival of embryos with spontaneous cleft lip exposed to 6-aminonicotinamide has been reported in the A/J mouse (Goldstein *et al.*, 1965).

Another interesting feature was that the effect of antihistamines (diphenhydramine in particular) appeared only in the clefts with additional malformations, whereas the effect of antianxiety drugs (valium or diazepam in particular) appeared only in the cases of clefts without other malformations. The association with valium has now been reported in two other studies (Safra and Oakley, 1975; Aarskog, 1975), and is beginning to look convincing. However, it must be remembered that the relative increase in risk is probably only about four-fold (i.e., an absolute risk of 1 in 250), and that it is still not clear whether valium itself or some associated factor is at fault.

Another drug suspected of teratogenicity is diphenylhydantoin (Meadow, 1970; South, 1972; Loughnan *et al.*, 1973; Hill *et al.*, 1974), and here also the evidence is becoming impressive—not only for cleft lip but for a variety of other malformations. Evidence from a Montreal study (Dansky *et al.*, 1975) suggests that maternal epilepsy *per se* is not at fault, that barbiturates may also be implicated. The combination of diphenylhydantoin and barbiturates seems more teratogenic than either, singly. Hanson and Smith

(1975) have identified a "dilantin facies," which we have also noted, though it is not particularly consistent or distinctive.

The uterine environment has been shown to be important in many of the experimental teratogens where it has been looked for (Biddle and Fraser, 1977), and in spontaneous cleft lip in the mouse (Davidson *et al.*, 1969; Bornstein *et al.*, 1970). One attempt to demonstrate such an effect in man was negative, but if the same mating pattern had been used in the experimental studies they would probably also have failed to show the effect. Studies of population differences (Leck, 1972) and interracial crosses (Ching and Chung, 1974) give little evidence of significant environmental factors, maternal or cultural (Burdi *et al.*, 1972).

To turn, now, to the question of genetically determined predisposing factors in man, it is interesting to note some evidence in support of the multifactorial threshold hypothesis discussed at the beginning of this paper. The data for cleft lip and/or cleft palate and (with occasional discrepancies) for cleft palate fit the criteria defined by Carter (1969) quite convincingly (Fraser, 1970).

The secondary palate closes later in female than in male human embryos (Burdi and Silvey, 1969), which is consistent with the higher frequency of cleft palate in females.

Another piece of evidence comes from the Finns, who have one of the highest incidences of cleft palate in any ethnic group. The width of the head increases from East to West, and so does the frequency of cleft palate (Saxen, 1975a), as predicted by this hypothesis. It is tempting to think that the (Pierre) Robin syndrome results from micrognathia inhibiting forward growth of the tongue. There are alternative explanations, however, and in the comparable syndrome in mouse embryos treated with vitamin A the micrognathia appears after the palate has closed (Shih *et al.*, 1974).

Measurements of facial topography in the parents of children with cleft lip and palate suggested certain statistical differences compatible with the face-shape hypothesis (Fraser and Pashayan, 1970), and these have been, in part, supported by cephalometric studies of near relatives and twins (Kurisu *et al.*, 1974), though cephalometry may not be the best approach to the kind of differences that prove to be relevant. It would be interesting to extend this type of study, using "physioprints" (Fraser and Pashayan, 1970) or some more sophisticated technique for measuring facial topography, in populations with a high frequency of cleft lip, such as the Japanese. Preliminary studies among the Japanese, done by Dr. M. Yasuda (Fraser and

Pashayan, 1970) and among British Columbia Indians (J. R. Miller, personal communication) supported the hypothesis, but sample sizes were too small to be statistically significant. However, considering the face shape studies in the mouse alluded to above, which suggest that the susceptible phenotype varies, depending on the mechanism of cleft lip formation, one should not expect a clear-cut association to emerge, and it is not suprising that the differences found are relatively small. Ideally, one might expect to see a clearer pattern by studying the relatives of children with cleft lip produced by a known teratogen (such as DPH), but the practical difficulties are formidable.

Another useful approach might be to study families in which a dominant gene causes cleft lip or cleft palate, or both, or neither, such as the lippit syndrome (Van der Woude, 1954). The facial topography might suggest why some individuals who carry the gene develop one or the other defect and some neither. We have some scattered observations in support of this.

Finally, we do not know what the relation is between face shape in the early embryo and in the postnatal individual. Studies of differences in embryonic face shape between populations with different frequencies of cleft lip could be useful here. Also, we need to know something of the inheritance of face shape, an almost unknown quantity at present.

In conclusion, the accumulation of data from experimental teratology, family studies, and epidemiological surveys are consistent with the multifactorial/threshold model for both cleft palate and cleft lip. Consideration of the complex systems involved, and the fact that all the specific factors identified so far have relatively small effects, suggests that, even if the sophisticated statistical techniques of Morton and others (Chung *et al.*, 1974; Elson and Yelverton, 1975) cannot distinguish between multifactorial and major gene-with-modifier models for the common types of cleft lip and cleft palate, the real biological systems are truly multifactorial.

REFERENCES

Aarskog, D. 1975. Association between maternal intake of diazepam and oral clefts. *Lancet* **II**: 920.

Biddle, F. G., and Fraser, F. C. 1977. Maternal effects in experimental teratology, *In* Wilson, J. G., and Fraser, F. C. (Eds.), *Handbook of Teratology*, vol. II. Plenum Press, Philadelphia, U.S.A.

Bingle, G. J., and Niswander, J. D. 1975. The absence of a maternal effect in human cleft lip and palate. *Am. J. Dis. Child.* **27**(6): 18A

Bonner, J. J., and Slavkin, H. C. 1975. Cleft palate susceptibility linked to histocompatibility (H–2) in the mouse. *Immunogenetics* **2**: 213–218.

Bornstein, S., Trasler, D.G., and Fraser, F. C. 1970. Effect of the uterine environment on the frequency of spontaneous cleft lip in CL/Fr mice. *Teratology* **3**(4): 295–298.

Burdi, A. R., and Silvey, R. G. 1969. Sexual differences in closure of the human palatal shelves. *Cleft Palate J.* **6**(1): 1–7.

Burdi, A., Feingold, M., Larsson, K. S., Leck, I., Zimmerman, E. F., and Fraser, F. C. 1972. Etiology and pathogenesis of congenital cleft lip and cleft palate, an NIDR State of the Art Report. *Teratology* **6**(3): 255–270.

Carter, C. O. 1970. Multifactorial inheritance revisited. *In* Fraser, F. C., and McKusick (Eds.), *Congenital malformations*. Excerpta Medica, New York, U.S.A., pp. 227–232.

Ching, G. H. S., and Chung, C. S. 1974. A genetic study of cleft lip and palate in Hawaii. I. Interracial Crosses. *Am. J. Hum. Genet.* **26**: 162–176.

Chung, C. S., Ching, G. H. S., and Morton, N. E. 1974. A genetic study of cleft lip and palate in Hawaii. II. Complex segregation analysis and genetic risks. *Am. J. Hum. Genet.* **26**: 177–188.

Dansky, L., Andermann, E., Andermann, F., and Sherwin, A. 1975. Major congenital malformations in the offspring of epileptic women. *Am. J. Hum. Genet.* **27**(6): 31A.

Davidson, J. G., Fraser, F. C., and Schlager, G. 1969. A maternal effect on the frequency of spontaneous cleft lip in the A/J mouse. *Teratology* **2**(4): 371–376.

Elston, R. C., and Yelverton, K. C. 1975. General models for segregation analysis. *Am. J. Hum. Genet.* **27**: 31–45.

Erickson, R. P. 1975. Differentiation, alloantigens, histocompatibility loci and birth defects. *Am. J. Hum. Genet.* **27**(4): 554–557.

Fraser, F. C. 1969. Gene-environment interactions in the production of cleft palate. *In* Nishimura, H., and Miller, J. R. (Eds.), *Methods for teratological studies in experimental animals and man*. Igaku Shoin Ltd., Tokyo. pp. 34–49.

Fraser, F. C. 1970. The genetics of cleft lip and cleft palate. *Am. J. Hum. Genet.* **22**(3): 336–352.

Fraser, F. C. 1974. Some aspects of maternal effects on congenital malformations. *In* Janerich, D. W., Skalko, R. G. and Porter, I. H. (Eds.), *Congenital defects: New directions in research*. Academic Press, New York, U.S.A., pp. 17–22.

Fraser, F. C. 1976. Relation of animal studies to the problem in man. *In* Wilson, J. G., and Fraser, F. C. (Eds.), *Handbook of teratology*. Plenum Press, Philadelphia, U.S.A.

Fraser, F. C., and Pashayan, H. 1970. Relation of face shape to susceptibility to congenital cleft lip: A preliminary report. *J. Med. Genet.* **7**(2): 112–117.

Goldstein, M. B., Fraser, F. C., and Roth, Katherine. 1965. Resistance of A/Jax mouse embryos with spontaneous congenital cleft lip to the lethal effect of

6-aminonicotinamide. *J. Med. Genet.* **2**(2): 128–130.

Hanson, J. W., and Smith, D. W. 1975. The fetal hydantoin syndrome. *J. Pediat.* **87**: 285–290.

Hay, S. 1967. Incidence of clefts and parental age. *Cleft Palate J.* **4**: 205–213.

Hill, R. M., Verniaud, W. M., Horning, M. G., McCulley, L. B., and Morgan, N. F. 1974. Infants exposed in utero to antiepileptic drugs. *Am. J. Dis. Child.* **127**: 645–653.

Kurisu, K., Niswander, J. D., Johnson, M. C., and Mazaheri, M. 1974. Facial morphology as an indicator of genetic predisposition to cleft lip and palate. *Am. J. Hum. Genet.* **26**: 702–714.

Leck, I. 1971. Further tests of the hypothesis that influenza in pregnancy causes malformations. *HSMHA Health Rep.* **86**: 265–269.

Leck, I. 1972. The etiology of human malformations: insights from epidemiology. *Teratology* **5**(3): 303–314.

Long, S. Y., Larsson, K. S., and Lohmander, S. 1973. Cell proliferation in the cranial base of A/J mice with 6-AN-induced cleft palate. *Teratology* **8**: 127–138.

Loughnan, P. M., Gold, H., and Vance, J. C. 1973. Phenytoin teratogenicity in man. *Lancet* **I**(7794): 70–72.

Meadow, S. R. 1970. Congenital abnormalities and anticonvulsant drugs. *Proc. R. Soc. Med.* **63**: 48–49.

Morton, N. E., Yee, S., Elston, R. C., and Lew, R. 1970. Discontinuity and quasi-continuity: Alternative hypothesis of multifactorial inheritance. *Clin. Genet.* **1**: 81–94.

Perry, T. B., and Fraser, F. C. 1972. Paternal age and congenital cleft lip and palate. *Teratology* **6**(2): 241–246.

Safra, M. J., and Oakley, G. P. 1975. Association between cleft lip with or without cleft palate and prenatal exposure to diazepam. *Lancet* **II**(7933): 478–480.

Saxen, I. 1975. Etiological variables in oral clefts. *Proc. Finnish Dent Soc.* **71** (Supp. 3): 1–40.

Saxen, I. 1975. Epidemiology of cleft lip and palate. *Br. J. Prev. Soc. Med.* **29**: 103–110.

Schultz, A. H. 1920. The development of the external nose in whites and negroes. *Carnegie Inst. of Wash., Contributions to Embryology* **9**: 173–190.

Shih, L. Y., Trasler, D. G., and Fraser, F. C. 1974. Relation of mandible growth to palate closure. *Teratology* **9**: 191–202.

South, J. 1972. Teratogenic effect of anticonvulsants. *Lancet* **II**(7787): 1154.

Trasler, D. G. 1965. Strain differences in susceptibility to teratogenesis: Survey of spontaneously occurring malformations in mice. *In* Wilson and Warkany (Eds.), *Teratology*. U. Chicago Press, Chicago, U.S.A., pp. 38–55.

Trasler, D. G. 1968. Pathogenesis of cleft lip and its relation to embryonic face shape in A/J and C57BL mice. *Teratology* **1**(1): 33–49.

Trasler, D. G., and Leong, S. 1976. Embryonic face shape in mice with induced and inherited cleft lip. *Teratology* (in press).

Van der Woude, A. 1954. Fistula labii inferioris congenita and its association with cleft lip and palate. *Am. J. Hum. Genet.* **6**(2): 244–256.

Verrusio, A. C. 1970. A mechanism for closure of the secondary palate. *Teratology* **3**(1): 17–20.

Zimmerman, E., Babiary, B. S., and Allenspach, A. L. 1975. Ultrastructural evidence of contractile systems in mouse palates prior to rotation. *Dev. Biol.* **47**(1): 32–44.

DISCUSSION

Recurrence Rate in Offspring and Siblings of Patients with Cleft Lip and/or Cleft Palate

Hideo Koguchi and *Hideo Tashiro*

The recurrence rates in offspring and siblings of patients with cleft lip and cleft palate in two surveys in our oral surgery clinic at Kyushu University are presented.

In the first survey, reported previously by Fujino *et al.* (1967), questionnaires were sent by post to parents of a total of 928 patients who visited our clinic from 1922 to 1952.

In the second survey (Koguchi, 1975), questionnaires were sent to parents of 2,519 patients who visited the clinic afterwards.

According to the combined data of the both surveys, the recurrence rate in offspring of the cleft lip propositi with or without cleft palate was estimated to be 2.33 percent, and that of the cleft palate alone was 1.61 percent (Table 1).

As a result of the second survey, the recurrence rate in siblings of the cleft lip propositi whose parents were both unaffected was 1.84 percent, and that of the cleft palate alone was 2.33 percent (Table 2).

As is seen in Table 3, if one parent was affected, the rate among siblings was 15.79 percent for cleft lip. No such family was recorded in the cleft

TABLE 1. Recurrence rate in offspring of the propositi.

	Propositi		Children					
Type	Sex	Those having offspring	Males Total	affected (%)	Females Total	affected (%)	Both sexes Total	affected (%)
CL+CLCP	Male	114	126	3 (2.38)	123	2 (1.63)	249	5 (2.01)
	Female	99	100	2 (2.00)	80	3 (3.75)	180	5 (2.78)
	Both	213	226	5 (2.21)	203	5 (2.46)	429	10 (2.33)
CP	Male	21	29	2 (6.90)	28	0 (0.00)	57	2 (3.51)
	Female	29	35	0 (0.00)	32	0 (0.00)	67	0 (0.00)
	Both	50	64	2 (3.13)	60	0 (0.00)	124	2 (1.61)

Cl: Cleft lip CLCP: Cleft lip with cleft palate
CP: Cleft palate

Department of Oral Surgery, Faculty of Dentistry, Kyushu University, Fukuoka, Japan.

TABLE 2. Recurrence rate in siblings of patients whose parents were both non-affected.

Propositi			Brothers		Sisters		Both	
Type of abnormality	Sex	No.	Total	affected (%)	Total	affected (%)	Total	affected (%)
CL+CLCP	Male	367	471	12 (2.55)	471	6 (1.27)	942	18 (1.91)
	Female	269	389	7 (1.80)	355	6 (1.69)	744	13 (1.75)
	Both	636	860	19 (2.21)	826	12 (1.45)	1686	31 (1.84)
CP	Male	42	56	2 (3.57)	43	0 (0.00)	99	2 (2.02)
	Female	105	168	3 (1.79)	119	4 (3.36)	287	7 (2.44)
	Both	147	224	5 (2.23)	162	4 (2.47)	386	9 (2.33)

TABLE 3. Recurrence rate of cleft lip and/or cleft palate in siblings of propositi with positive family histories.

Affected relatives of propositi	Type of propositi	Siblings: Total no.		Affected		%	
i) Parent	CL	2	19	1	3	50.00	15.79
	CLCP	17		2		11.76	
	CP	—		—		—	
ii) One or more sibs	CL	36	65	2	4	5.56	6.15
	CLCP	29		2		6.90	
	CP	26		2		7.69	
iii) Second-degree relative	CL	54	70	1	3	1.85	4.29
	CLCP	16		2		12.50	
	CP	20		4		20.00	
iv) Third-degree relative	CL	35	70	1	2	2.86	2.86
	CLCP	35		1		2.86	
	CP	17		0		0	

palate group. If both parents were unaffected but at least one more sibling was affected, the rate in siblings excluding one affected sibling was 6.15 percent for cleft lip and 7.69 percent for cleft palate. If both parents were also unaffected but a second-degree relative of the propositus—that is, uncle, aunt, grandparent, nephew, or niece—was affected, the rate was 4.29 percent for cleft lip and 20 percent for cleft palate. If a third-degree relative—that is, great-grandparent, great-uncle, great-aunt, or first cousin—was affected, the rate was 2.86 percent for cleft lip, and no affected sibling was found in the cleft palate group.

In Table 4 it is seen that, if a fourth-degree relative was affected, the rate was 2.33 percent for cleft lip, and no such family was recorded in the

TABLE 4. Recurrence rate of Cleft lip and/or cleft palate in siblings of propositi with positive family history.

Affected relatives of propositi	Type of propositi	Siblings					
		Total no.		Affected		%	
v) Fourth degree relative	CL	19	43	0	1	0	2.33
	CLCP	24		1		4.17	
	CP	—		—		—	
vi) Fifth degree relative	CL	7	22	0	0	0	0
	CLCP	15		0		0	
	CP	2		0		0	
vii) More remote relative	CL	10	34	0	0	0	0
	CLCP	24		0		0	
	CP	5		0		0	

cleft palate group. If a fifth-degree or more remote relative was affected, none of 56 siblings of cleft lip patients and 7 siblings of cleft palate patients showed cleft.

Thus, the recurrence rate in siblings of propositi is higher in familial cases than in sporadic cases. If secondary cases are known among relatives, the closer their relationship with the propositi is, the more the recurrence rate in the siblings is increased.

REFERENCES

Fujino, H., Tashiro, H., Sanui, Y., and Tanaka, K. 1967. Empirical genetic risk among offspring of cleft lip and cleft palate patients. *Jap. J. Human Genet.* **12**: 62–68.

Koguchi, H. 1975. Recurrence rate in offspring and siblings of patients with cleft lip and/or cleft palate. *Jap. J. Human Genet.* **20**: 207–221.

Genetics of Common Diseases

C. O. Carter

Conventional measures of public health applied to the whole population, such as clean water supplies, adequate nutrition, and the control of infection, have had no influence on the incidence of two groups of common conditions: congenital malformations, such as the facial clefts, the neural tube malformations, and the congenital heart malformations; and common constitutional disorders of adult life such as schizophrenia and coronary artery disease. The reason for this is likely to be that there is a substantial genetic component in their etiology as well as an environmental component. To prevent these disorders, it seems likely that we must first learn to recognize those genetically at risk and then learn how to protect those at risk from the additional environmental factors.

It is a feature of these conditions that they show a degree of familial aggregation—that is, an increased risk to relatives over the risk in the general population, which it is difficult to explain purely by common family environment, but which also does not fit any simple monogenic pattern of inheritance. A large sample of patients with such conditions will usually be found to be heterogeneous, including perhaps a small fraction with a purely environmental causation (for example, congenital heart malformation following intrauterine infection with rubella) and a small fraction simply monogenically determined, as for example the dominant syndrome of mucous pits of the lower lip in association with cleft lip and palate, or the monogenic form of hyperbetalipoproteinaemia in association with coronary artery disease. The majority of cases, however, particularly isolated cases of the malformation unaccompanied by other abnormalities, are clearly determined in a more complex fashion.

One of the best illustrations is provided by the cleft lip, with or without

MRC Clinical Genetics Unit, Institute of Child Health, London, England.

TABLE 1. Family studies in cleft lip (±cleft palate), showing proportion of relatives affected.

Relatives	Copenhagen, 1942	Utah, 1963, 1971	London, 1965	Copenhagen, 1971
Sibs	56/1140 (4.9%)	63/1574 (4.0%)	25/774 (3.2%)	36/931 (3.9%)
Children	— —	7/164 (4.3%)	17/565 (3.0%)	18/513 (3.5%)
Aunts and uncles	43/5343 (0.8%)	31/4747 (0.7%)	14/2476 (0.6%)	— —
Nephews and nieces	— —	7/832 (0.8%)	7/1021 (0.7%)	— —
First cousins	19/7703 (0.2%)	42/11698 (0.4%)	7/3518 (0.2%)	— —

cleft palate, which I will hereafter call the cleft lip malformation. The proportion of monozygotic co-twins affected is not yet precisely established, but is probably of the order of 40 percent, compared with about 5 percent of dizygotic co-twins affected. The findings in three large studies in Caucasian populations for first, second, and third degree relatives are shown in Table 1 (Fogh-Anderson, 1942; Woolf *et al.*, 1963; Woolf, 1971; Carter, 1965). In each of these populations, the birth frequency in the general population is about one per thousand live-births. The main features of the family patterns shown are: the proportion of children affected is as high as the proportion of sibs affected (hence even modified recessive inheritance is excluded); the sharp diminution in the proportion of relatives affected as one passes from monozygotic co-twins to first-degree, to second-degree, and to third-degree relatives. The diminution is about ten-fold, seven-fold, and two-and-a-half-fold, respectively.

It is also noteworthy that the proportion affected of second-degree relatives is much the same, six to eight per thousand, though uncles and aunts and nephews and nieces are born two generations, perhaps 50 years or more, apart. This indicates that the intrauterine environmental influences concerned must be constant over many years.

This and similar family patterns are explicable by many models, but the two simplest are additive polygenic with a threshold (illustrated in Figure 1) and much modified monogenic inheritance, with most patients heterozygous for the mutant gene involved but most such heterozygotes being unaffected. The distinction between the two hypotheses becomes blurred where, on the modified monogenic hypothesis, the factors influencing the manifestation rate in heterozygotes are at least in part genetic. The argument then becomes

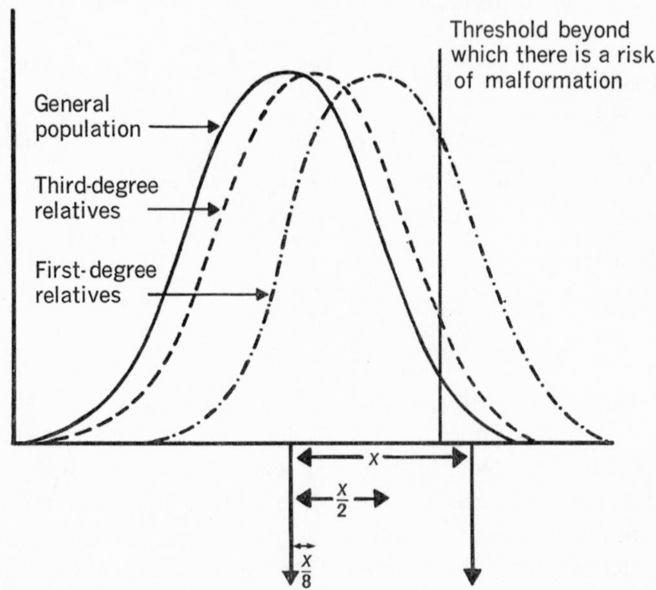

FIG. 1. Normally distributed polygenic predisposition with a threshold.

whether variation at one gene locus is making a major contribution to the development of the condition. It is noteworthy too that on the additive polygenic model it is only necessary to assume that polymorphism at a few gene loci is involved. Two common alleles at each of four or five gene loci would give an approximately normal distribution of the genetic predisposition to develop the malformation.

Additional features that best fit the polygenic model are:

1) *An effect of severity.* It is reasonable to suppose on the polygenic model that the more severe degrees of the malformation are the more extreme deviants from the population mean. In the case of the cleft lip malformation, the risk to sibs is decreased to about 2 percent where the index patient has a unilateral cleft lip alone and increased to about 6 percent where this patient has bilateral cleft lip and palate (Carter, 1965; Fraser, 1970).

2) *An effect of sex.* It is reasonable to suppose on the model that

patients of the sex more rarely affected are more extreme deviants. The sex ratio is too close to unity for the cleft lip malformation for this to be seen clearly, though there is a suggestion of such an effect (Woolf, 1971). In the case of pyloric stenosis, however, with a male: female sex ratio of 4: 1, the risk to first-degree relatives of female index patients is three times higher than that to relatives of male index patients (see below).

3) *An effect of having a first-degree relative of the index patient already affected.* With polygenic inheritance, parental couples will have a continuous spectrum of risk of having an affected child, from a very low risk to a high risk where the mid-parental value for the genetic predisposition is close to the threshold. Where parents have already had two affected children, they will tend to be among those with a relatively high risk. Similarly, where one or the other parent is her/himself affected, the mean parental predisposition will tend to be high. In the case of the cleft lip malformation, in both situations the risk to further children appears to be of the order of 12 percent.

One further feature of polygenic inheritance is that a small parental consanguinity effect is to be expected, since parental consanguinity involves a degree of assortative mating, a genotypic correlation of 0.125, for any polygenic predisposition.

The other common single malformations; the neural tube malformations (anencephaly and spina bifida); the common heart malformations (patent ductus arteriosus, ventricular septal defect, pulmonary stenosis); the common skeletal malformations (congenital dislocation of the hip, talipes equinovarus) also show, insofar as data are available, family patterns similar to those for the cleft lip malformation. Data for the sibs and

TABLE 2. Proportion of sibs and children of index patients with pyloric stenosis who were also affected.

Relatives	Male index patients		Female index patients	
	London	Belfast	London	Belfast
Brothers	21/546 (3.8%)	52/544 (9.6%)	25/273 (9.2%)	20/160 (12. %)
Sons	19/347 (5.5%)	—	20/106 (18.9%)	—
Sisters	15/565 (2.7%)	13/428 (3.0%)	10/263 (3.8%)	6/159 (3.8%)
Daughters	8/337 (2.4%)	—	7/100 (7.0%)	—

children of index patients with pyloric stenosis (Carter and Evans, 1969; Dodge, 1970) are summarized in Table 2. Data for sibs of index patients with neural tube malformations (Carter *et al.*, 1968; Carter and Evans, 1973) are summarized in Table 3, and the first data coming through on the risks to the children of the few surviving patients with spina bifida cystica (Tünte, 1971; Carter and Evans, 1973; Laurence, personal communication) are summarized in Table 4. Data for sibs and children of patients with congenital dislocation of the hip are summarized in Table 5 (Carter and Wilkin-

TABLE 3. Proportion of sibs of index patients with central nervous system malformations who were also affected.

Locality	Birth frequency in population (%)		Proportion of sibs affected	Percentage of sibs affected
South Wales	Spina bifida	0.41	52/854	5.2
	Anencephaly	0.35	29/709	
London	Spina bifida	0.15	25/730	4.4
	Anencephaly	0.14	41/754	

TABLE 4. Numbers of children of index patients with central nervous system malformations who were also affected.

Locality	Index patients		Number of children	
			Total	Affected
Munster	Fathers	4	8	2
	Mothers	6	18	0
London	Fathers	18	45	1
	Mothers	47	78	2
South Wales	Fathers	7	15	0
	Mothers	9	15	3
Total		91	179	8

TABLE 5. Proportion of sibs and children of index patients with congenital dislocation of the hip who were also affected.

Relatives	Male index patients		Female index patients	
	London	Edinburgh	London	Edinburgh
Brothers	6/104	0/61	1/200	4+3*/369
Sons	0/19	0/3	0/48	0+3*/51
Sisters	9/134	4+1*/53	7/183	18+13*/376
Daughters	2/25	0/4	5/45	3+9*/66

* Signifies neonatal diagnosis

son, unpublished; Wynne-Davies, 1970). There is a complication here: since the introduction of methods of diagnosing the condition in the neonatal period, the ascertained incidence of the condition has increased from about one per thousand to about four per thousand births in Western Europe. Clearly three out of the four neonateally ascertained patients would have recovered spontaneously. In estimating risks to relatives in twins of the old "late" diagnosis, it is appropriate to divide the neonatal cases by four. The data on midline cleft palate are perhaps less suggestive of polygenic inheritance and more of heterogeneity, with some cases due to modified monogenic inheritance and many cases with little genetic determination.

The data for sibs and children for two series of congenital heart malformations are summarized in Table 6 (Nora *et al.*, 1970; Zetterquist, 1972).

The additive polygenic model was much improved by Falconer's (1965) concept of regarding the x-axis as representing the total liability, both genetic and environmental. It is now reasonable to regard the threshold as an absolute cut-off level beyond which all individuals are affected and not merely at risk of malformation. This is illustrated in Figure 2. Further, this concept made possible a rough estimate of the "heritability" of the condition in the particular population studied, using "heritability" in the sense of the fraction of the total variance of the liability to develop the malformation that is due to additive genetic variation. Smith's improvement (1970) takes account of the fact that, where the distribution of the liability in the population is normal, this will not be the case in close relatives, especially monozygotic twins. For example, for cleft lip malformation, the birth frequency in the population and the proportion of first, second, and

TABLE 6. Proportion of sibs and children of index patients with congenital heart disease who were also affected.

Type of malformation	Location	Sibs	Children
Patent ductus arteriosus	Texas	17/505 (3.4%)	4/117 (3.4%)
	Uppsala	17/663 (2.6%)	18/490 (3.7%)
Ventricular septal defect	Texas	24/543 (4.4%)	6/162 (3.7%)
Atrial septal defect	Texas	11/342 (3.2%)	5/190 (2.6%)
	Uppsala	6/633 (0.9%)	6/397 (1.5%)
Pulmonary stenosis	Texas	10/345 (2.9%)	3/102 (2.9%)
Coarctation of the aorta	Texas	5/272 (1.8%)	— —
	Uppsala	5/283 (1.8%)	5/191 (2.6%)
Transposition of the great vessels	Texas	4/209 (1.9%)	— —

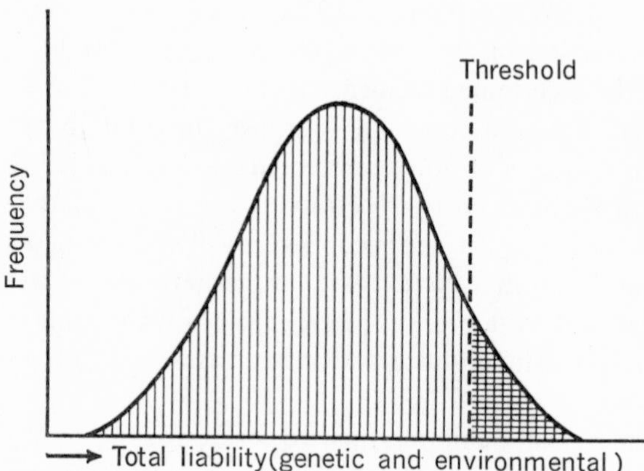

FIG. 2. Falconer's model of polygenic inheritance.

third-degree relatives affected implies correlations between index patient and relatives of approximately 0.9, 0.45, 0.20, and 0.09 for MZ twins, first, second, and third-degree relatives, respectively. The respective theoretical correlations with additive polygenic inheritance are 1.0, 0.5, 0.25, and 0.125. If there were no influence of common family environment, the family data would imply "heritabilities" of 0.9, 0.9, 0.8, and 0.7 for MZ co-twins, first, second, and third-degree relatives, respectively. There will be a common family environment, and it is plausible to suppose that the true "heritability" is perhaps 0.6 and that the correlation is progressively increased with closer relationship by an increasing degree of common family environment. The data for pyloric stenosis imply correlations of about 0.40 for brothers of male patients and 0.45 for sisters of female patients, suggesting upper limits of heritability of 0.8 and 0.9 respectively. For the neural tube malformations, the correlations implied between sib and index patient are 0.33 in the South Wales series and 0.40 in the London series, giving upper limits of heritability of 0.7 and 0.8.

Turning now to some of the common diseases of adult life: family studies of these diseases involve difficulties in diagnosis and in correcting for age of onset which do not apply with congenital malformations; nevertheless, similar family patterns are often indicated. In the case of the major psychoses, schizophrenia and manic-depressive psychosis, the lifetime risk of developing each disorder is so high—about 1 percent in Britain with British criteria of diagnosis (Slater and Cowie, 1971)—that there is little to choose between polygenic and modified monogenic models in fitting the family patterns found. The proportion of sibs found affected in most series is about 8 percent; of children, rather more, 10–12 percent; of uncles, aunts, nephews and nieces, and grandchildren, about 2.5 percent; and, a bit anomalously, of first cousins, also about 2.5 percent (Zerbin-Rudin, 1967). It is interesting now that small series are coming through for children of schizophrenic mothers who have been adopted and separated from their mothers at birth and nevertheless still apparently have a 10 percent risk (Heston, 1966). Family data for coronary artery disease (Slack and Evans, 1966), rheumatoid arthritis, diabetes mellitus, coeliac disease, and ankylosing spondylitis (Emery and Lawrence, 1967) are also suggestive of a multifactorial etiology, including polygenic inheritance.

One must emphasize that the concept of polygenic inheritance is essentially a useful descriptive model, and estimates of heritability are, in my opinion, not without value in planning further studies; where high, they imply that preventive measures will need to be selectively applied to those genetically at risk, though this will not necessarily be the case. Tuberculosis will be prevented by total elimination of the tubercule bacillus, even though the heritability of pulmonary tuberculosis may be substantial. On the other hand, it would be unreasonable to abandon wheat as an article of diet because some 1 per cent of the population in northwest Europe are at risk of developing coeliac disease if they eat wheat.

The aim must be to define the individual gene loci involved and the individual environmental triggers involved. In the case of coeliac disease, the main environmental trigger is wheat gluten, and the HLA B locus is making some genetic contribution, since 85 percent of patients in Britain but only 25 percent of the general population have this gene. In the case of ankylosing spondylitis, the HLA B gene locus, or, more probably, a gene-locus very closely linked to it, is a stronger and major source of genetic variation in liability. Some 7 percent of western Europeans have the HLA B_{27} allele, but this is found in 90 percent of patients with ankylosing spondylitis (Brewerton, 1975). Nevertheless, this implies that only about 5 percent of men and about 0.5 percent of women with this gene develop overt clinical disease. These remarkable and somewhat unexpected findings serve to encourage us that we may be able to identify before long other gene-loci making substantial contributions to the variation in liability to develop congenital malformations and common diseases.

REFERENCES

Brewerton, D. A. (Ed.) 1975. Symposium on histocompatibility and rheumatic disease. *Ann. Rheum. Dis.* Suppl.

Carter, C. O. 1965. The inheritance of common congenital malformations. *Prog. Med. Genet.* **4**: 59–84.

Carter, C. O., David, P. A., and Laurence, K. M. 1968. A family study of major central nervous system malformations in South Wales. *J. Med. Genet.* **5**: 81–106.

Carter, C. O. and Evans, K. 1969. Inheritance of congenital pyloric stenosis. *J. Med. Genet.* **6**: 233–254.

Carter, C. O., and Evans, K. 1973. Spina bifida and anencephalus in Greater London. *J. Med. Genet.* **10**: 209–304.

Carter, C. O., and Evans, K. 1973. Children of adult survivors of spina bifida cystica. *Lancet* **II**: 924–926.

Dodge, J. A. 1970. Infantile hypertrophic pyloric stenosis (thesis for MD degree). University of Wales.

Emery, A. E. H., and Lawrence, J. S. 1967. Genetics of ankylosing spondylitis. *J. Med. Genet.* **4**: 239–244.

Falconer, D. S. 1965. The inheritance of liability to disease. *Ann. Hum. Genet.* **29**: 51–76.

Fogh-Andersen, P. 1942. *Inheritance of hare lip and cleft palate.* Busck, Copenhagen, Denmark.

Fraser, F. C. 1970. The genetics of cleft lip and palate. *Am. J. Hum. Genet.* **22**: 336–352.

Heston, L. L. 1966. Psychiatric disorders in foster home reared children of schizophrenic mothers. *Br. J. Psych.* **112**: 819–825.

Nora, J. J., McGill, C. W., and McNamara, D. G. 1970. Empiric recurrence risks in common and uncommon congenital heart lesions. *Teratology* **3**: 325–329.

Slack, J., and Evans, K. A. 1966. The increased risk of death from ischaemic heart disease in first degree relatives of 121 men and 96 women with ischaemic heart disease. *J. Med. Genet.* **3**: 239–257.

Slater, E., and Cowie, V. 1971. *The genetics of mental disorders.* Oxford University Press, London, England.

Smith, C. 1970. Heritability of liability and concordance in monozygotic twins. *Ann. Hum. Genet.* **34**: 85–91.

Tünte, W. 1971. Fortflanzungsfähigkeit, heiratshäufigkeit und zahl und beschaffenheit der nackkommen bei patienten mit spina bifida sperta. *Humangenetik* **13**: 43–48.

Woolf, C. M., Woolf, R. M., and Broadbent, T. R. 1963. A genetic study of cleft lip and palate in Utah. *Am. J. Hum. Genet.* **15**: 209–215.

Woolf, C. M. 1971. Congenital cleft lip: a study of 496 propositi. *J. Med. Genet.* **8**: 65–83.

Wynne-Davies, R. 1970. A family study of neonatal and late-diagnosis congenital dislocation of the hip. *J. Med. Genet.* **7**: 315–333.

Zerbin-Rudin, E. 1967. Endogen psychosen in humangenetik, ein Kurzes Handbuck V/2. Ed. Becker, P. E. Georg Thieme Verlag, Stuttgart, Germany.

Zetterquist, P. 1972. *A clinical and genetic study of congenital heart defects.* University of Uppsala, Sweden.

DISCUSSION 1

Indirect Inguinal Hernia: A Multifactorial Threshold Trait

Ei Matsunaga

As reviewed by Dr. Carter, evidence has been accumulating that a number of common developmental abnormalities are likely to be inherited as the result of a polygenic predisposition, with a threshold beyond which individuals are at risk. I should like to present some of our recent data (Sawaguchi *et al.*, 1975; Matsunaga *et al.*, 1975) to show that indirect inguinal hernia may probably be another example.

Indirect inguinal hernia is very common among children. For obvious anatomical and developmental reasons, boys are prone to the condition, and if they are affected on one side, it is more often on the right than on the left side. Although postnatal factors such as excessive physical exertion may be involved in the manifestation of hernia, it is generally recognized that the principal cause is the existence of a congenital sac resulting from failure in closure of the tunica vaginalis.

Table 1 represents the distribution of our probands by sex and laterality of hernia. They are 1,723 in number; all were operated on at the National Children's Hospital in Tokyo; about 88 percent of them were under 5 years of age at the time of the operation. There is a marked preponderance of male probands, the ratio of males to females being 2.8: 1. In both sexes cases of bilateral hernia account for 20 percent, the remaining 80 percent

TABLE 1. Distribution of probands with indirect inguinal hernia, by sex and laterality (Sawaguchi *et al.*, 1975).

Sex		Laterality of hernia			Total
		Right	Left	Bilateral	
Males	No.	588	431	254	1,273 (73.9%)
	%	46.2	33.9	20.0	
Females	No.	177	184	89	450 (26.1%)
	%	39.3	40.9	19.8	
				Total	1,723 (100%)

Department of Human Genetics, National Institute of Genetics, Mishima, Japan.

TABLE 2. Incidence of inguinal hernia among parents and elder siblings, relative to that in the general population (Sawaguchi *et al.*, 1975).

Probands		Fathers	Elder brothers	Mothers	Elder sisters
Males	Unilat.	×3.3	×3.6	×3.1	×4.0
	Bilat.	×4.1	×3.8	×6.4	×9.2
	Total	×3.5	×3.6	×3.9	×5.3
Females	Unilat.	×4.4	×2.9	×5.3	×6.6
	Bilat.	×4.9	×5.9	×11.1	×8.8
	Total	×4.5	×3.4	×6.6	×7.1
Incidence in the general population		0.042	0.085	0.015	0.038

being of unilateral hernia. The 80 percent is divided equally by dextral and sinistral cases in the female probands, while in the male probands there are more dextral than sinistral cases.

Table 2 gives the incidence of inguinal hernia among parents and elder siblings of the probands, relative to that in the general population. The data are based on information obtained from parents concerning past affliction of inguinal hernia. The control data are those reported by Kajimoto *et al.* (1974), who made an extensive survey by questionnaire of about 160,000 school children. The control figures for the siblings are the incidences of boys and girls who gave a positive history of inguinal hernia, including relatively mild cases in which the condition had undergone spontaneous cure; since the figures were based on answers of the parents, they may be comparable with our siblings' data. On the other hand, the control figures for the fathers and the mothers are the incidences of boys and girls who had been operated on, for most of our parents who gave a positive answer may be regarded as those cases that had been operated on; parents in whom spontaneous cure had taken place in early childhood were, for lack of memory, likely to have given a negative answer.

From the family pattern shown in the table, two features are readily apparent that fit well the hypothesis of polygenic inheritance with a threshold. First, the relative incidence of hernia among parents and siblings tended to be higher, by about 20–50 percent, if the proband was of the more rarely affected sex (that is, a female) than if it was a male. Second, the relative incidence tended to be higher, though slightly, if the condition in the proband was more severe (that is, bilateral) than if it was unilateral. In particular, the relative incidence tended to be about 50–100 percent greater if the proband was a female affected with bilateral hernia than if it was a male with unilateral hernia. Incidentally, there was no indication of an increase in parental consanguinity in our data. Using Falconer's procedure (1965), the heritability of liability to indirect hernia was estimated at 64 ± 3 percent from the regression coefficients of parents on probands.

Finally, as a by-product of our study, it has been found that our probands contained more twins than would have been expected, 1.2 percent as against 0.5 percent in the general population. This finding supports Bakwin's (1971) observation that "presumably twins are especially prone to indirect inguinal hernia, owing to a developmental delay in closure of the tunica vaginalis."

In conclusion, indirect inguinal hernia appears to be determined by polygenic inheritance with threshold. The threshold is generally higher in girls than in boys, but it is lowered if intrauterine development is delayed.

REFERENCES

Bakwin, H. 1971. Indirect inguinal hernia in twins. *J. Pediat. Surg.* **6**: 165–168.

Falconer, D. S. 1965. The inheritance of liability to certain diseases, estimated from the incidence among relatives. *Ann. Human Genet.* **29**: 51–76.

Kajimoto, T., Nakamura, S., Furuta, Y., and Kawaguchi, R. 1974. On the incidence and spontaneous cure of indirect inguinal hernia in Japanese children. *Shoni-Geka* **6**: 513–521 (in Japanese).

Matsunaga, E., Sawaguchi, S., and Honna, T. 1975. Estimation of heritability of liability to indirect inguinal hernia. *Jap. J. Human Genet.* **20**: 197–200.

Sawaguchi, S., Matsunaga, E., and Honna, T. 1975. A genetic study on indirect inguinal hernia. *Jap. J. Human Genet.* **20**: 187–195.

DISCUSSION 2

Family Studies of Systemic Lupus Erythematosus, A Late-Onset Disease of Lower Incidence

Toshiyuki Yanase, K. Kajiyama and Masaya Yamaguchi

Dr. Carter has referred to common diseases with frequencies of at least 1 in 1,000, but we would like to call your attention to the late-onset diseases with incidences lower than these.

Family data on the late-onset diseases of relatively lower incidence have not been collected as extensively as those for common malformations and other common diseases of adult life such as ischemic heart disease. Systemic lupus erythematosus is a representative example of such diseases. Analyses of such a disease involve more difficulties because of the lower incidence in the general population, extreme deviation in sex ratio, and more complex process in the development of morbid conditions, etc. Nevertheless, the family patterns of systemic lupus erythematosus appear similar to those in some congenital malformations interpreted as being of "threshold character," and the analyses of gene-environment interactions would also be profitable in the etiology and prophylaxis of the disease.

Systemic lupus erythematosus, usually abbreviated as "SLE," is a disease entity characterized by pathologic changes in the collagenous tissues which affect the vascular system, skin, and serous and synovial membranes. As a major feature of this entity, the autoimmune mechanism has recently been an important issue. In addition, this disease is extremely frequent in females, about 12 times more than males, especially between 10 and 40 years of age. We have just mentioned above that this disease is uncommon in general, but today it is not infrequently encountered in major clinical institutions. For instance, 15 cases of SLE are among about 60 patients now hospitalized in our clinic.

1. Recurrence risk among the first-degree relatives of SLE patients

In the general population, incidences ranging from 5 to 130 per million have been reported. However, these values cannot be used immediately for the analysis concerned, because they represent only an approximation for

First Department of Medicine, Faculty of Medicine, Kyushu University, Fukuoka, Japan.

a population comprising both sexes and all age groups, neonatal to adult old period. Therefore, we have attempted to approximate the incidence on the basis of other sources of information.

According to a nationwide investigation conducted by the "Japanese Research Organization on SLE" in the past three years, the number of female patients precisely diagnosed based upon the ARA Diagnostic Criteria was approximately 8,300 in the entire country of Japan (Table 1). According to the Report on Vital Statistics, the number of females aged 10 to 40 living in Japan in 1974 was about 26,000,000. From these numbers, the incidence of SLE among females of this group may tentatively be estimated to be at least 1 in 3,200.

Now, let us estimate the recurrence among relatives of SLE patients.

A number of families in which more than two members were affected with SLE have been reported in the medical literature. These involve mostly sister-sister and mother-daughter combinations, including an extreme instance of four affected sisters. In most family studies, however, the degree of relationship of families included in the calculation is not clear. Therefore, we would like to present our recent data, though it is only preliminary material based on a survey still in progress.

In our studies, three definite, one probable, and one possible SLE have been found among 184 first-degree relatives aged 10 to 40 of 74 propositi. These were carefully judged based on the ARA Diagnostic Criteria (Figure 1). Thus, the risk to the first-degree female relatives was estimated to be 0.0163

TABLE 1. Incidence in the control population and recurrence among relatives of SLE patients.

Incidence of SLE in the control population	
Population of females aged 10–40 in Japan (1974)	26,457,000
Number of affected females registered (a minimum estimate)	8,308
Incidence	.000314 (1/3,185)

Recurrence among the first-degree relatives			
Subjects: 184 relatives aged 10–40 of 74 propositi			
Classification	Number	Rate (Q)	$\sqrt{p}$
Definitely affected relatives	3	.0163	
Definitely and probably affected relatives	4	.0217	.0177
Definitely, probably, and possibly affected relatives	5	.0272	

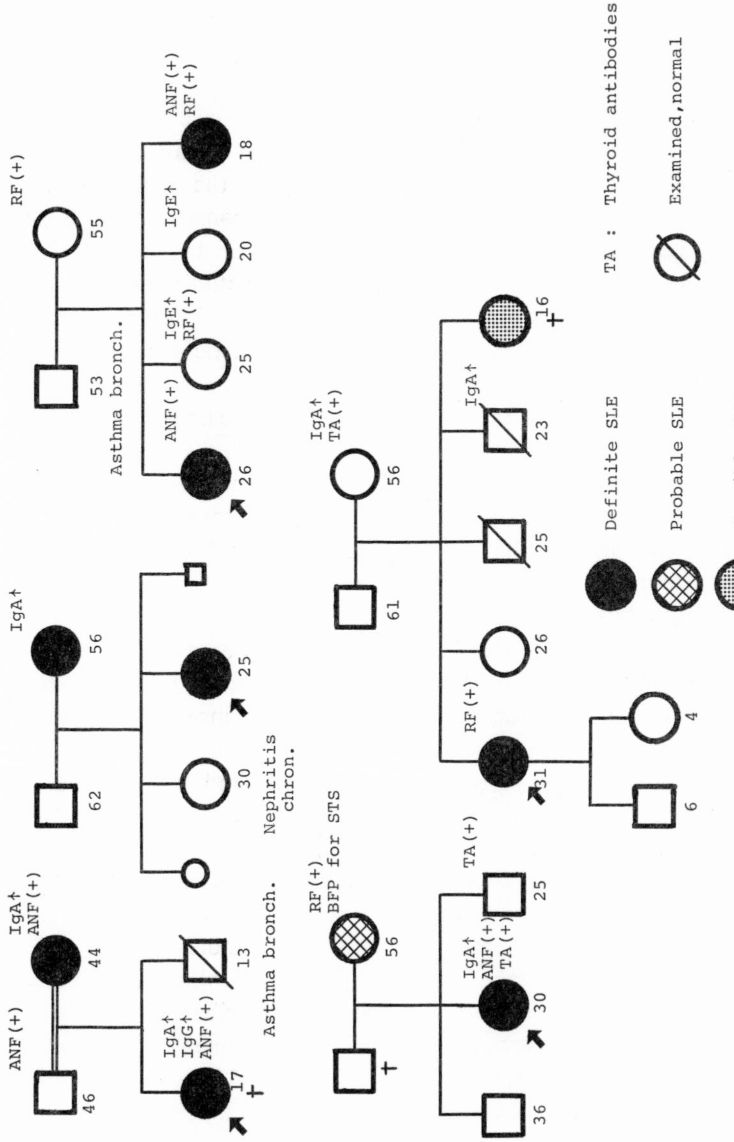

FIG. 1. Families in which more than two members were affected with SLE (the present study).

when three definitely affected relatives were marked, 0.0217 when three definitely and one probably affected relative were marked, and 0.0272 when five definitely to possibly affected relatives were marked (Table 1). A comparison of these rates with the incidence in the control population shows that the first-degree relatives of the propositi have about 51 to 87 times the risk to the controls. It may be noted that no affected case has been detected so far among unrelated cohabitants in the same family.

Needless to say, there still remain problems in considering SLE as a clear-cut model of multifactorial inheritance similar to some common malformations usually ascertained at birth. Further studies are needed to test whether the liability underlying the development of SLE is under the control of a polygenic system. However, if the genetic predisposition is additive polygenic, the square root of the population incidence would be expected to reflect more or less the recurrence rate in the first-degree relatives of the propositi in accordance with Edwards' formula. As shown in Table 1, the expected value calculated on this assumption does not appear to depart much from the observed values. In the present investigation we have subjected individuals aged 10 to 40 to the analysis, but plan to employ in the future a more narrow range of age, say 10 to 20, and make some corrections for the data to be obtained.

In passing, the rate of consanguineous marriages among parents of 79 patients is 4.2 percent, which does not differ significantly from that in the general population, and the reproductive performance of the affected individuals is not much reduced despite the fulminating manifestations of immunological aberration in their prereproductive and reproductive ages and the long-term administration of steroid hormones.

2. Level of serum immunoglobulins in the SLE and control relatives

Disorders presumably due to the autoimmune mechanism and unusual immunological reactions in serum and tissues are more frequent among 450 relatives of SLE patients compared with control relatives, though further efforts are needed to match sex and age distributions between the two groups. It may be particularly noted that rheumatoid arthritis and polyarthralgia of unknown etiology are found in 6.2 percent of female relatives of SLE patients. These findings are in close agreement with those obtained by Leonhardt (1964, 1967) and Larsen (1972).

Figure 2 shows the frequency distributions for the serum immunoglobulins. The mean levels and variances of Ig G and Ig A are significantly

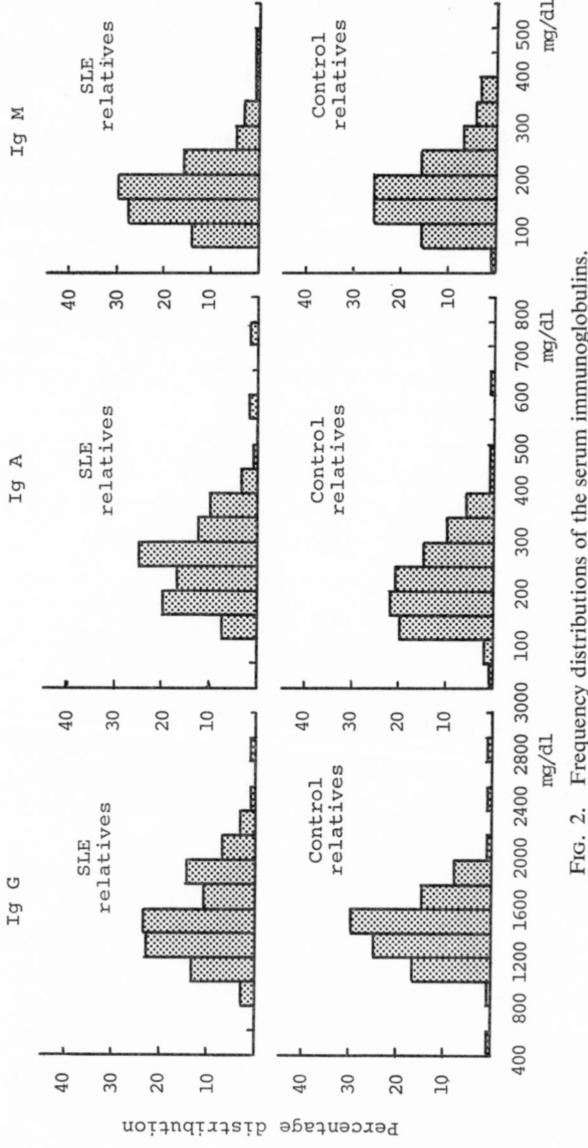

FIG. 2. Frequency distributions of the serum immunoglobulins.

greater in the SLE relatives than in the control relatives with a more marked skewness to the right. Ig M, however, shows no significant difference between the two groups, though the level in females is higher than in males.

Estimates of heritability of immunoglobulins were tentatively computed from the linear regression of offspring to parent and the sib-sib correlation. In the control relatives, correlation coefficients between sibs were 0.45 for Ig A and 0.56 for Ig M, and those between parent and offspring were 0.33 for Ig A and 0.25 for Ig M. For all types of immunoglobulin, sib correlations are higher than parent-offspring correlations, suggesting that heritability based on sibs is inflated by environmental and/or dominance variation common to full sibs. In the SLE relatives, on the other hand, correlation coefficients between parent-offspring are of the order of 0.25 for all types of immunoglobulin, and those between sibs are nearly 0. This may be attributable to the higher incidence of hyperimmunoglobulinemia among the SLE relatives. In contrast to these, the correlation coefficient between parents is fairly high, being 0.37.

From these results obtained in the control relatives, heritability in the narrow sense was estimated to be 0.66 for Ig A and 0.50 for Ig M, though these figures are very tentative at the present time.

REFERENCES

The Ministry of Welfare 1974. *Proc. of Group Researches on Systemic Lupus Erythematosus*, ed. by the Ministry of Welfare, 1975.

Leonhardt, T. 1964. *Acta Med. Scand.*, Suppl.: 416.

Leonhardt, T. 1967. *Clin. Exp. Immunol.* **2**: 743.

Larsen, R. A. 1972. *Acta Med. Scand.*, Suppl.: 543.

The Multifactorial Model of Liability in Familial Disease: Methods, Applications, and Limitations

Charles Smith

SYNOPSIS

The multifactorial model of disease liability has proved a useful tool in studying familial disease in man and in animals. The model allows us to express data on disease frequencies in the population and in relatives of affected individuals in terms of correlations among relatives, and to interepret these using the standard statistics of quantitative genetics, the heritability and the genetic correlation. These parameters are independent of the population frequency and of the type of relative studied, both of which had an overriding effect on most of the statistics previously used in the field. The model has been able to account for several apparent paradoxes in familial data, such as low concordance rates in monozygous twins for diseases considered to have an important genetic component. Its uses include the estimation of recurrence risks from family histories and other data, the prediction of disease frequencies in future generations, the discrimination between different modes of inheritance, and the testing for genetic heterogeneity in familial disease. The model is flexible and can be extended to data with three or more classes (of variable size), and so can deal with many kinds of ordinal data met in study of normality and of abnormality in man and animals. An extensive review of much of the recent work with the model has been given by Curnow and Smith (1975).

THE MODEL

In the multifactorial model it is assumed that there are a large number of factors, both genetic and environmental, and each with a small effect,

---

A.R.C. Animal Breeding Research Organisation, Edinburgh, Scotland.

contributing to an underlying liability to a disease (Falconer, 1965). Since there are many factors with small effects, the distribution will be continuous and there will always be a transformation which could (conceptually, since it is not required in practice) transform it to a normal distribution. Thus the model can use all the convenient properties of the normal curve and all the genetic theory for normally distributed continuous traits. While the theory strictly requires a large number of small effects, in practice, with as few as 5–10 factors, the distribution becomes continuous and the model should fit quite well, except in extreme cases. Of course the number of factors is usually not known in practice for any continuous trait, yet the theory has given good approximations to observed data and proved very productive in prediction and in application, for example in animal genetics.

With the underlying continuous liability scale for phenotype, it is convenient to define a threshold value. Above this level, all individuals are affected, or manifest the trait, while any below the threshold level are unaffected. The more severely affected the individual, the higher his liability is estimated to be, so that the model allows for variable severity (Reich, James, and Morris, 1972) and similarly for variable age at onset (Falconer, 1967). The abrupt threshold has been queried by clinicians and criticized as being biologically unsound (Edwards, 1969). However, its definition and use are for simplicity and for statistical conveninence, for it has been shown (Smith, 1971a) that the threshold corresponds exactly to a normal distribution of *genetic* liability, with a cumulative normal risk function. This is biologically much more acceptable and realistic.

Since affected individuals have a high liability, exceeding the threshold, their relatives will also tend to have a higher liability than average, and they will have a higher than average frequency of the disease. Thus, from the frequency of the disease in the population and the raised frequency in relatives of affected individuals, the correlation in liability between relatives can be estimated. This can be done in several ways using the properties of the normal curve—by regression (Falconer, 1965; Reich, James, and Morris, 1972) or by numerical integration (Smith, 1970)—or the properties of the bivariate normal curve, by the tetrachoric correlation (Edwards, 1969). The three later methods allow for a reduced variance in the liability distribution of relatives of affected individuals and so avoid a slight bias in the original Falconer (1965) method.

Common Familial Environment

The next step is to interpret the correlation in liability between relatives into a genetic framework. In making a genetic interpretation, this step is crucial, for it is essential to eliminate or discount any possible common familial environmental effects among relatives, or else these will seriously bias the estimates of the genetic parameters. This can be done by using the correlations estimated from relatives living apart or of unrelated individuals living together, so as to adjust the correlations for relatives living together. Often data from such groups may be limited and special searches may have to be made. Several recent studies on special collected data sets for schizophrenia (Heston, 1966; Rosenthal, 1970; Schulsinger, 1972) illustrate well the value of the approach in resolving the effects of nature and nurture in familial disease. On the other hand, if common familial environmental effects are not discounted, the whole genetic interpretation will be suspect.

Heritability of Liability

Using the theory of quantitative genetics (e.g., Falconer, 1964), the correlation (r) in liability between relatives can be interpreted in terms of the heritability of liability (h^2) by

$$r = Rh^2$$

where R is the genetic relationship between the relatives. The heritability is a measure of the proportion of the total variation in liability which is additively genetic—that is, which is transmissible to the next generation. Thus the heritability is the basic genetic parameter in summarizing observations among relatives and for making predictions with the multifactorial model.

Estimates of heritability of liability have now been made for a large number of familial disorders (Smith, 1975). In general, many of the conditions have high heritability estimates, mostly from 40–80 percent, indicating that genetic variation is important in the variance in liability to these conditions. However, most of the estimates must still be regarded as tentative since familial environmental effects have been properly discounted in only a few of the studies. Conditions which manifest themselves later in life or have a variable age at onset tend to have lower heritability estimates, as might be expected from the accumulating effects of different environments between individuals. Usually, as in other species, there is good agreement in heritability estimates in different locations and in different populations. However, there is no prior reason why this should be so. The estimates of heritability refer to variation *within* populations, and strictly give no information about genetic differences *between* populations. Although the estimates are independent of the frequency of the disease in the population studied, they do depend on the level of ascertainment of affected individuals (Smith, 1974).

The multifactorial model was successful in accounting for several apparent paradoxes in data on familial disease. For example, the sex with the lower disease frequency usually has the higher frequency of affected relatives (of both sexes). This was shown to be expected with the liability model, because there was a higher threshold for the sex with the lower disease frequency, and so affected individuals of that sex have a higher average liability. Falconer (1965) and Carter (1969) applied these results to pyloric stenosis and to other disorders. Another paradox was the low *proband* concordance rates found in monozygous (MZ) twins for many diseases thought to have a high genetic component. It was shown (Smith, 1970) that if the population frequency is low, then the MZ concordance rate will also be low, even at quite high levels of heritability. This is becaue an individual with a high genetic liability (as shown by his affected MZ co-twin) still has only a low probability of exceeding the phenotypic threshold, for to do so requires a large (random) environmental deviation effect.

A common misconception is that if heritability is high then environmental factors can have only small effects. This is true with the current set of environmental factors. But if conditions change or novel environmental factors are brought into play, then there can be a large shift in mean liability and so in the frequency of the disease. The same is true for highly heritable continuous traits such as height, where the average has increased with improved nutrition, and the proportion of individuals over a certain height (the threshold) is now larger than in previous generations. A high heritability suggests that there are no important environmental factors in the current set, so that in research and treatment, novel environmental factors and treatments should be looked for.

Other Forms

The model can also be applied to normal all-or-none traits such as handedness (Annett, 1973) and can be extended from the (0, 1) form to deal with multiple classes both in normality and in abnormality (Reich, James, and Morris, 1972). Its use should then be appropriate for the genetic analysis of familial data on ordinal scores used in many fields, such as psychology and psychiatry. An iterative maximum likelihood genetic method, using the liability model, has been developed to analyze genetic data with any number of classes and with classes of variable size (Bradley, Sales, and Smith, 1976).

The liability model, in a different form, has long been used in animal genetics for the analysis of threshold (0, 1) traits (Robertson and Lerner, 1949). The analysis is usually done on the (0, 1) scale, and the transformation to the normal scale has come later, whereas in the form of the model used here the transformation is made initially. Assessment of the biases in estimates of the parameters using the (0, 1) data directly have been made through simulation by several authors (Van Vleck, 1972; Olausson and Ronningen, 1975).

Application

The heritability estimate, with its standard error, summarizes data on familial frequencies for a disease. It allows the testing for differences between estimates from different types of relatives and from different regions or populations. If there are significant differences the reasons for them can be explored, and if not, the estimates can be combined into a single figure, summarizing all the evidence from a number of studies. Thus real differences will be highlighted and studied while trivial differences are dismissed and replaced by a single parameter.

Another application of the heritability is in the prediction of the future frequency for a condition, following a change in the fitness of affected individuals. Since the prediction deals with the mean genetic liability, it must be assumed that environmental conditions are unchanged. Another difficulty is that it is not known whether the condition is in equilibrium or is changing over time. The change in frequency can be predicted from the change in average liability due to the change in reproductive fitness of affected individuals. However, the simple method proposed by Holloway and Smith (1975) turned out to underestimate the expected change. This method did not take account of the bias in the original Falconer (1965) heritability estimates and in the reduction in variance after loss of affected individuals. When these effects are allowed for, then good estimates of the net change in frequency are obtained. This was confirmed using a simple method proposed by Matsunaga (1976), that the frequency in the next generation can be estimated from the two-way table

		Males	
		Normal	Affected
Females	Frequency	$(1-P)/T$	fP/T
Normal	$1-P/T$	P_0	P_1
Affected	fP/T	P_1	P_2

$T = fP + (1 - P)$

where P is the population frequency, P_0, P_1, and P_2 are the frequencies in offspring of matings with 0, 1, and 2 affected parents, and f is the reproductive fitness of affected individuals. For example, take a condition with $P=P_0=1$ percent, $P_1=5$ percent, and $P_2=20$ percent. If the initial fitness $f_1=0$, (a lethal), and $f_2=1$ (due to a new treatment giving a complete cure), then net change in population frequency in the next generation would be about 8 percent. If $f_1=10$ percent and $f_2=50$ percent, the net change would only be about 3 percent.

Matsunaga (1976) extended his method to further generations and concluded for a case with $P=P_0$ that the frequency will not continue to increase but will reach a plateau or new equilibrium at just above the frequency found in the first generation after relaxation of selection. His result depends on the assumption that the frequency of affected individuals from different mating types will be constant over time. However, we do not know what these frequencies will be and so cannot use Matsunaga's method for further generations. The conclusion of a plateau is rather unlikely since any forces previously acting to raise the frequency of the condition will no longer be balanced if selection is relaxed. However, it can be shown by the liability model (Smith, Matsunaga, and Holloway, 1976) that with the same changes in fitness, approximately the same net changes in frequency will be obtained in each subsequent generation. However, this prediction concerns the *net* change due to genetic effects, and not the absolute change due to genetic and environmental effects. In practice, it may never be possible to test the genetic predictions made, because it will usually not be possible in man to separate genetic and non-genetic effects and trends.

Recurrence Risks

In simple Mendelian disorders, the mode of inheritance is known, and recurrence risks can be derived from genetic theory, even for complex family histories and with additional information on associated traits (Heuch and Li, 1972; Conneally and Heuch, 1974). For non-Mendelian conditions, empiric (observed) risks are often used rather than risks derived from any theory. These measure average risks for all families rather than applying to a particular counselling case, and do not take into account other factors affecting risk such as age, sex, severity, mortality, and associated traits (Darlow, Smith, and Duncan, 1973). A method to derive risks with the multifactorial model was given by Smith (1971a). This can take account of differences in frequency between sexes and of differences in liability and heritability due to variable severity and age of onset. A computer program RISKMF (Smith 1972) is also available for use in genetic counselling.

In additional to family history, there may also be information on a continuous trait associated with the disease which is useful in risk estimation, such as glucose tolerance level in diabetes and blood pressure in hypertension. A method was developed (Smith and Mendell, 1974) to use such information on an individual and on his relatives in estimating recurrence risks of the disease, and again a computer program was written to perform the operations. However, it turned out that this is only likely to be useful in certain circumstances: when the correlation of liability and the trait is intermediate or when the trait cannot be measured on the individual himself, for example, if he were too young, or not yet born.

Discrimination of Genetic Models

A basic dilemma in familial disease is whether liability is really multifactorial or if there are one or more loci with *major* effects on the condition. The strategy for research and treatment might be quite different if the underlying genetic form were known. So this is a question which always gives rise to considerable controversy and research effort. It was hoped that analysis of data on familial frequencies from different types of relatives and of data on segregation within sibships would allow a statistical solution of the problem. Unfortunately, as predicted by Edwards (1960), it was shown (Smith, 1971b; Kruger, 1973) that discrimination between different modes of inheritance is very difficult indeed, except in rather extreme situations. These attempts used two extreme models on simulated data, namely the single locus, two-allele modes with variable penetrance and environmental cases, compared with the multifactorial model. If discrimination is difficult for these extreme models, then it will be even more difficult for intermediate models. Data from second- and third-degree relatives is theoretically more useful in discrimination (Van Regermorter and Smith, 1976), but unfortunately it is usually much less reliable than data on first-degree relatives. One advantage of the multifactorial model is that it uses fewer parameters; only two, the population frequency and the heritability, compared with three or four in the single locus model, the gene frequency, and the proportion of each genotype affected.

With variable penetrance the single locus model also could be said to become "multi-" factorial, for it implies that there are other genetic and environmental factors affecting liability. Several authors such as Elston and Campbell (1971) and Kidd and Cavalli-Sforza (1973) have shown that single locus models with variable penetrance can account for observed familial and segregational data in familial diseases quite as well as the multifactorial model does. However, the levels of penetrance invoked tended to be rather low, often less than 10 percent. They also suggested that the heritability of liability is of doubtful value. Their model (with three genotypes), in some data on schizophrenia, found that only 10–15 percent of the total variation in liability was due to differences between genotypes, whereas the heritability was 80 percent in the same data. However, their low estimate of genetic variance arose from the low estimated frequency of the extreme genetic class and not from small estimated differences between the genotypes. That is, their estimate of genetic variation depended on the frequency of the disease. Their model also assumes no genetic variation in penetrance, which is biologically unlikely.

It is interesting to note that even with plants and animals there has been little genetic resolution of major loci in continuous traits. This is despite the large amount of genetic research on economic traits and the complex facilities for control, special matings, and experimentation. More recently, MacLean, Morton, and Lee (1975) have developed methods which may allow resolution of any major effects (defined as more than one standard deviation in liability between extreme genotypes) if these exist. However, the methods are much less sensitive for discontinuous (0, 1) traits than for continuous traits, since much less information is available in the (0, 1) data.

Genetic Heterogeneity

Genetic heterogeneity has proved common among Mendelian clinical disorders. It is likely also to be common in non-Mendelian familal conditions, as improved clinical and laboratory techniques become available to classify different types. The multifactorial model can be used to test for genetic heterogeneity among subsets of the disease, whether these are defined clinically, biochemically, physiologically, or statistically. Distinct subsets can be easily identified by differential frequencies of types among relatives; otherwise the genetic correlation (Falconer, 1967) provides a good measure of genetic equivalence (Smith, 1976). For example, no clear discrimination was found between early and late onset diabetes, and a genetic correlation of 0.65 between their respective liabilities was calculated. On resolution of a disease into distinct subsets, the estimates of heritability of the subsets may well be higher (not lower as Edwards (1969) suggests) than the estimate for the original disease. Conversely, if two diseases, such as spina bifida and anencephaly, are analyzed separately, the individual heritability estimates are lower than the estimate from the combined data, indicating that effectively they represent the same genetic disease.

Major Loci

Individual loci with large effects have been shown recently to be important in several non-Mendelian familial disorders. These are discussed elsewhere in the symposium by Carter. The genes concerned have turned out to have rather low penetrance and moderate frequencies. Unfortunately the associations have been found only after extensive testing of a large number of loci and conditions, rather than through a logical link. Moreover, they follow upon a decade of unimportant or negative results on tests of association of diseases with a large number of other loci. No doubt further important associations will be found in the future, and it is interesting to speculate about how many of the common non-Mendelian familial disorders will be resolved in this way. Moreover, since true multifactorial inheritance can never be proven, there are likely always to be attempts to detect major loci involved in unresolved familial diseases.

One consequence of finding loci with abnormal genotypes having low levels of penetrance is that the penetrance level puts an upper limit on recurrence risk. This contrasts with multifactorial inheritance where the risk continues to rise with increasing severity and family history. To this extent, the mode of inheritance would be important in risk estimation (van Regermorter and Smith, 1976) and so modifies previous conclusions (Smith, 1972) that the choice of model had little effect on the recurrence risk estimates.

LINKAGE

Another technique in resolving multifactorial inheritance has been to look for linkage between a marker locus and a locus for the disease or continuous trait, so as to identify and locate individual loci (Haseman and Elston, 1972; Hill, 1975; Smith, 1975). However, these methods depend on very close linkage with genes of major effect, else they have very little power in analysis (Robertson, 1973). In general the methods are unlikely to be of much value in resolving familial diseases.

DISCUSSION

The main value of the multifactorial model has been as a statistical tool to summarize data on frequencies of familial disease into standard and interpretable genetic statistics. The results for different relatives, different populations, and different diseases can be couched in the same form and so are more easily undertstood genetically and compared. The model had also been useful in resolving anomalies, predicting risks, resolving heterogeneity, predicting trends, and showing how difficult it is to discriminate between different models of inheritance. There have been two common misuses. One is to state that inheritance *is* multifactorial when this can never be proven. The other is to imply that, with high hertitability, environmental factors must *always* have small effects, when other new effects and other environmental factors may greatly affect the frequency of the condition.

In many respects the multifactorial model, with its two parameters, is very simplistic; nature is likely to be much more complex and heterogenous in its form and action. With intensifying research, separate entities in familial disease are continually being identified and isolated. Thus the multifactorial model may well be only a temporary tool in an explorative period, and will eventually be relegated to deal with the residual variation in liability after any major factors have been identified and their effects removed. How long this process will take and to what extent it will proceed are questions which hold the answer to the relevance and the utility of the multifactorial model in the future.

REFERENCES

Annett, M. 1973. Handedness in families. *Ann. Hum. Genet.* **37**: 93.

Bradley, J. S., Sales, D. I., and Smith, C. 1976. Estimation of heritaiblity of liability from ordinal data by maximum likelihood. (In prepration).

Carter, C. O. 1969. Genetics of common disorders. *Br. Med. Bull.* **25**: 52.

Conneally, P. M., and Heuch, I. 1974. A computer program to determine genetic risks: A simplified version of PEDIG (Heuch and Li, 1972). *Am. J. Hum. Genet.* **26**: 773.

Curnow, R. N., and Smith, C. 1975. Multifactorial models for familal diseases in man. *J. R. Stat. Soc. A.* **138**: 131.

Darlow, J. M., Smith, C., and Duncan, L. J. P. 1973. A statistical and genetical study of diabetes. III. Empiric risks to relatives. *Ann. Hum. Genet.* **37**: 157.

Edwards, J. H. 1960. The simulation of Mendelism. *Acta. Genet. Stat. Med.* (Basel) **10**: 63.

Edwards, J. H. 1969. Familial predisposition in man. *Br. Med. Bull.* **25**: 58.

Elston, R. C., and Campbell, M. A. 1970. Schizophrenia: Evidence for the major gene hypothesis. *Behav. Genet.* **1**: 3.

Falconer, D. S. 1964. *Introduction to quantitative genetics.* Oliver and Boyd, Edinburgh, Scotland.

Falconer, D. S. 1965. The inheritance of liability to certain diseases estimated from the incidence in relatives. *Ann. Hum. Genet.* **29**: 51.

Falconer, D. S. 1967. The inheritance of liability to diseases with variable age of onset, with particular reference to diabetes. *Ann. Hum. Genet.* **31**: 1.

Haseman, J. K., and Elston, R. C. 1972. The investigation of linkage between a quantitative trait and a marker locus. *Behav. Genet.* **2**: 3.

Heston, L. L. 1966. Psychiatric disorders in foster home reared children of schizophrenic mothers. *Br. J. Psych.* **112**: 819.

Heuch, I., and Li, F. H. F. 1972. PEDIG—A computer program for calculation of genotype probabilities using phenotype information. *Clin. Gen.* **3**: 501.

Hill, A. 1975. Quantitative linkage: A statistical procedure for its detection and estimation. *Ann. Hum. Genet.* **38**: 439.

Holloway, S. M. 1975. Effects of medical and social practices on the frequency of deleterious genes in the population. Unpublished Ph. D. Thesis, Edinburgh.

Holloway, S. M., and Smith, C. 1975. Effects of various medical and social practices on the frequency of genetic disorders. *Am. J. Hum. Genet.* **27**: 614.

Kidd, K. K., and Cavalli-Sforza, L. L. 1973. An analysis of the genetics of schizophrenia. *Soc. Biol.*, **20**: 254.

Kruger, J. 1973. Discrimination between multifactorial inheritance with threshold effect and two-allele single-locus hypothesis. *Humangenetik*, **17**: 181.

MacLean, C. J., Morton, N. E., and Lew, R. 1974. Analysis of family resemblance. IV. Operational characteristics of segregation analysis. *Amer. J. Hum. Genet.* **27**: 365.

Matsunaga, E. 1976. Possible genetic consequences of relaxed selection against common disorders with complex inheritance. *Hum. Genetik* **31**: 53.

Olausson, A., and Ronningen, K. 1975. Estimation of genetic parameters for threshold characters. *Acta. Agric. Scand.* **25**: 201.

Van Regermorter, N., and Smith, C. 1976. The importance of determining the mode of inheritance for the estimation of recurrence risks. *J. Genet. Hum.* **24**: 49.

Reich, T., James, J. W., and Morris, C. A. 1972. The use of multiple thresholds in determining the mode of transmission of semi-continuous traits. *Ann. Hum. Genet.* **36**: 163.

Robertson, A. 1973. Linkage between marker loci and those affecting a quantitative trait. *Behav. Genet.* **3**: 389.

Robertson, A., and Lerner, I. M. 1949. The heritability of all-or-none traits: Viability of poultry. *Genetics* **34**: 395.

Rosenthal, D. 1970. *Genetic theory and abnormal behavior.* McGraw-Hill, New York, U. S. A., p. 127.

Schulsinger, F. 1972. Psychopathy, heredity and environment. *Int. J. Ment. Hlth*, **1**: 190.

Smith, C. A. B. 1975. A non-parametric test for linkage with a quantiative character. *Ann. Hum. Genet.* **38**: 451.

Smith, C. 1970. Heritability of liability and concordance in monozygous twins. *Ann. Hum. Genet.* **34**: 85.

Smith, C. 1971a. Recurrence risks with multifactorial inheritance. *Am. J. Hum. Genet.* **23**: 578.

Smith, C. 1971b. Discrimination between different modes of inheritance in genetic disease. *Clin. Genet.* **2**: 203.

Smith, C. 1972. Computer programme to estimate recurrence risks for multifactorial familal disease. *Br. Med. J.* **1**: 495.

Smith, C. 1974. Concordance in twins: Methods and interpretation. *Am. J. Hum. Genet.* **26**: 454.

Smith, C. 1975. Quantitative inheritance. *In* Fraser and Mayo, O., *Text book of human genetics*. Blackwell, Oxford, England.

Smith, C. 1976. Statistical resolution of genetic heterogeneity in familial disease. *Ann. Hum. Genet.* **39**: 381.

Smith, C., Matsunaga, E., and Holloway, S. 1976. Effects of relaxed selection in common familial disorders with complex inheritance. (In preparation).

Smith, C., and Mendell, N. R. 1974. Reccurrence risks from family history and metric traits. *Ann. Hum. Genet.* **37**: 275.

Van Vleck, L. D. 1972. Estimation of heritability of threshold characters. *J. Dairy Sci.* **55**: 218.

III ANIMAL MODELS OF COMMON DISEASES

Hypertensive Strains of the Rat

Yukio Yamori

Hypertension is one of the most common diseases in the adult population, and among cultured people it is the basis of stroke and myocardial infarction which often cause death. In Japan stroke has been the most frequent cause of death for the past 25 years. However, the causes of most cases of hypertension in man, roughly 90 percent, are unknown and are classified as "essential" or "primary" hypertension.

Recent progress in experimental studies on hypertension is mainly based on the exploitation of animal models for essential hypertension in man, including spontaneously hypertensive rats (SHR) (Okamoto and Aoki, 1963), genetically hypertensive rats (Smirk *et al.*, 1958), and salt-sensitive rats (Dahl *et al.*, 1962). Among them so far, spontaneously hypertensive rats have been regarded as the best animal models for hypertension research, because: (1) incidence of hypertension in this strain is 100 percent; (2) hypertension is very severe, frequently over 200 mmHg; (3) hypertensive cardiovascular diseases are observed in high incidence; and (4) hypertension in SHR is similar to essential hypertension in hemodynamic characteristics.

In the early 1960s, SHR were separated by selective inbreeding from one couple of rats of the Wistar-Kyoto colony with mild hypertension. They are now in the F_{38} generation and are maintained at our laboratory, genealogically classified into several substrains with different characteristics. From these we recently succeeded in the selective breeding of SHR which develop stroke (cerebral hemorrhage and/or infarction) spontaneously at a rate of over 80 percent, and we separated them as *stroke-prone SHR* (SHRSP) from SHR substrains with an incidence of stroke of less than 10 percent [*stroke-resistant SHR* (SHRSR)] (Okamoto, Yamori, and Naga-

Department of Pathology, Faculty of Medicine Kyoto University, Kyoto & Japan Stroke Prevention Center, Izumo, Japan

oka, 1974). Furthermore, in search of better models for atherogenesis, Yamori (1974) confirmed that selected SHR substrains were prone to develop hypercholesterolemia as well as arterial fat deposition within an extremely short period when fed on a high-fat-cholesterol (HFC) diet, and termed these "arterio lipidosis-prone rate (ALR)." Gene-environment interactions were observed in these models for hypertension, stroke, or atherogenesis.

Models for Hypertension

Hypertension and complications. SHR develop moderate to severe hypertension without any obvious organic lesions—that is, primary hypertension—in 100 percent of the population, and they later develop various hypertensive cardiovascular diseases. The main complications of hypertension in SHR are cerebrovascular lesions such as infarction or hemorrhage, myocardial lesions, and nephrosclerosis as in essential hypertension. Cardiac hypertrophy is the most common gross pathological finding and especially marked in SHR in the advanced stage. A typical macroscopical infarction with extensive fibrosis is sometimes observed in myocardium. Kidneys of SHR with a long-standing hypertension show typical nephrosclerosis, and anginonecrosis of arterioles is commonly observed histopathologically in SHR with severe hypertension. Therefore, the SHR is not only a model for hypertension but also a good model for hypertensive complications.

Heredity and environment. The fact that the SHR was established by selective inbreeding from among Wistar-Kyoto indicates the importance of heredity in the etiology of this hypertension. Moreover, the selection of this hypertensive strain was nearly completed in the first six generations (Okamoto, 1969). Therefore, it seemed that the number of major genes involved in this hypertension was relatively small. The mode of heredity was analyzed by cross-breeding between the SHR and the normotensive Wistar strain (Tanase, Suzuki, Ooshima, Yamori, and Okamoto, 1970). The distribution of blood pressure in various crossgenerations showed that the average blood pressure in F_1 hybrids was intermediate between the two parent strains, and the distributions of blood pressure in F_2 and the two backcross generations were continious with the means near the mid-parent values (Figure 1). These results indicated that the heredity of this hypertension was neither dominant nor recessive, but was multifactorial inheritance in an additive mode. Therefore, the number of major genes was estimated on the assumption of multifactorial inheritance of independent and equiv-

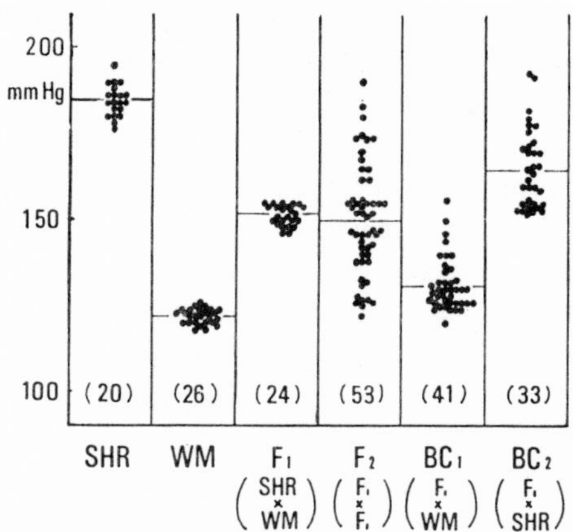

FIG. 1. Distribution of blood pressure in the males of various generations obtained by crosses between SHR and normotensive rats (WM: Wistar-Mishima).

alent genes. The minimum number of major genes calculated according to Wright's formula was unexpectedly small: two or three. Moreover, the degree of genetic determination of blood pressure analyzed from the variances in F_1 and F_2 generations was extremely high, from 86 to 96 percent. The conclusion of these genetic analyses was that hypertension in SHR is genetically determined to a large extent in an additive mode by a relatively small number of major genes plus an indefinite number of minor genes.

On the other hand, environmental factors and their interactions with genetic factors are also conceivable. Therefore, we observed the effect of extreme environmental conditions such as stress and diet on hypertension in SHR. Various stress loadings accelerated the development of hypertension, augmented the grade of hypertension, and also aggravated hypertensive cardiovascular lesions in SHR (Yamori, Matsumoto, Yamabe, and Okamoto, 1969). Extreme changes in dietary conditions, such as chronic excess salt intake, also clearly augmented the hypertension. However, salt excess is not indispensable for the development of hypertension, because SHR on low salt diets also developed and maintained hypertension (Aoki, Yamori, Ooshima, and Okamoto, 1972). This fact, again, indicates the greater importance of genetic disposition in the development of this hypertension.

Pathogenesis of spontaneous hypertension. The outline of the pathogenesis of spontaneous hypertension revealed up to the present can be briefly summarized as follows (Yamori, 1975): Under the genetic influence determined by a relatively small number of major genes, the metabolic deviation of the central nervous system results in the imbalance of central blood pressure regulation mechanisms, which tends to increase sympathetic outflow intrinsically or in response to environmental stimuli, because of the insufficiency of an inhibitory control mechanism. Thus, peripheral vascular resistance rises neurogenically in the initial stage. This increased pressure load enhances noncollagenous protein metabolism of arterial walls, which leads to medial hypertrophy—that is, "the adaptive structural vascular change" pointed out by Folkow in SHR as well as in essential hypertension (Folkow, Hallbäck, Lundgren, Sivertsson, and Weiss, 1973). On the other hand, the pressure load activates collagenous protein metabolism in arterial walls—that is, fiber formation which results in hypertensive arteriosclerosis (Yamori, 1974). Therefore, such a metabolic enhancement is a biochemical adaptation of vasculature to high pressure load; it precedes the structural changes in arterial walls and gradually increases the peripheral vascular resistance, the non-neural component of hypertension. Both of these adaptive metabolic and structural vascular changes seem to be the final common mechanisms of hypertension, whatever the primary causes may be, and hypertension is maintained by the increased peripheral vascular resistance. Such a consecutive relay from neural or any primary cause of hypertension to these final mechanisms is considered to be the main reason why neurogenically initiated labile hypertension is rapidly stabilized, or why the primary cause of hypertension has remained indistinct, especially in essential hypertension. The gene-environmental interaction seems to be important in both these initiation and maintenance mechanisms of hypertension.

A Unique Model for Stroke

Establishment of a model. Comparative studies on SHR and essential hypertension in man up to the present indicate a great similarity between them. However, the incidence of cerebrovascular lesions and of infarction or hemorrhage (so-called stroke) was relatively low, about 10 percent on the average before the F_{20} generation. Therefore, we attempted selective breeding of SHR which developed stroke spontaneously with a high frequency, and finally succeeded in establishing a strain of stroke-prone SHR

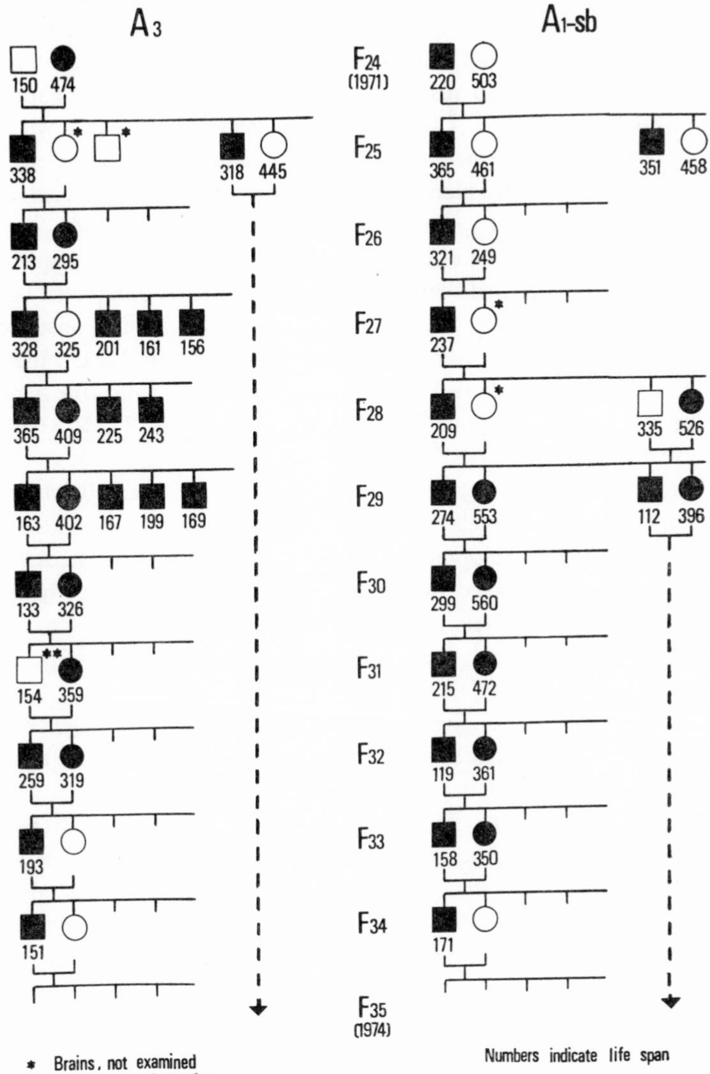

FIG. 2. Genealogical outline of selectively bred stroke-prone SHR (figures indicate life span).

in 1973 (Okamoto, Yamori, and Nagaoka). Because we could not breed the offspring from old SHR with definite signs of stroke, we selected some young candidates from the family with high incidence of stroke and mated as many of them as possible to obtain the offspring in advance. We maintained the offspring of SHR one or both parents of which died of stroke, and discarded the others. Thus we could selectively obtain the offspring of parents who had had strokes for the past 11 generations, as shown in the pedigrees in Figure 2. The incidence of stroke in adult males in the selectively bred offspring was greatly increased, from 39 percent to 83 percent on the average from the F_{27} to F_{32} generations. The selection effect was obvious, and the incidence of stroke after the F_{27} generation reached the maximum plateau level. So we decided that the selection was nearly completed because of other unavoidable deaths caused by pneumonia and so on. Consequently, these selectively bred SHR were named "stroke-prone SHR." On the other hand, we selectively maintained the offspring of SHR, in which the incidence of stroke was very low, about 7 percent on the average. These SHR were named "stroke-resistant SHR."

Symptoms and cerebral lesions. Stroke-prone SHR rapidly developed severe hypertension at a relatively young age in comparison with stroke-resistant SHR. The development of severe hypertension in stroke-prone SHR was somewhat delayed in females. They showed various symptoms such as irritability, paralysis (Figure 3 (a)), urinary incontinence, general weakness and attacks, and finally death at the average age of 9 and 13 months in males and females, respectively.

Autopsy revealed massive hemorrhage and softening in the telencephalon and also in the basal ganglia, which are the predilection sites of stroke in man (Figure 3 (b) and (c)).

Heredity and environment. The establishment of stroke-prone SHR indicated the importance of the genetic factor in the development of stroke. Genealogical studies showed that the incidence of stroke greatly increased in the offspring whose parents (one or both) had died of stroke for the preceding three generations. Moreover, the incidence of stroke became 100 percent in the offspring obtained by the crosses between two substrains of stroke-prone SHR, both of which had as high an incidence of stroke as 80 percent. These examples again substantiated the importance of the genetic factor in stroke. The mode of inheritance of stroke was analyzed by cross-breeding between stroke-prone and stroke-resistant SHR. F_1 and F_2 generations showed intermediate average blood pressure levels, and

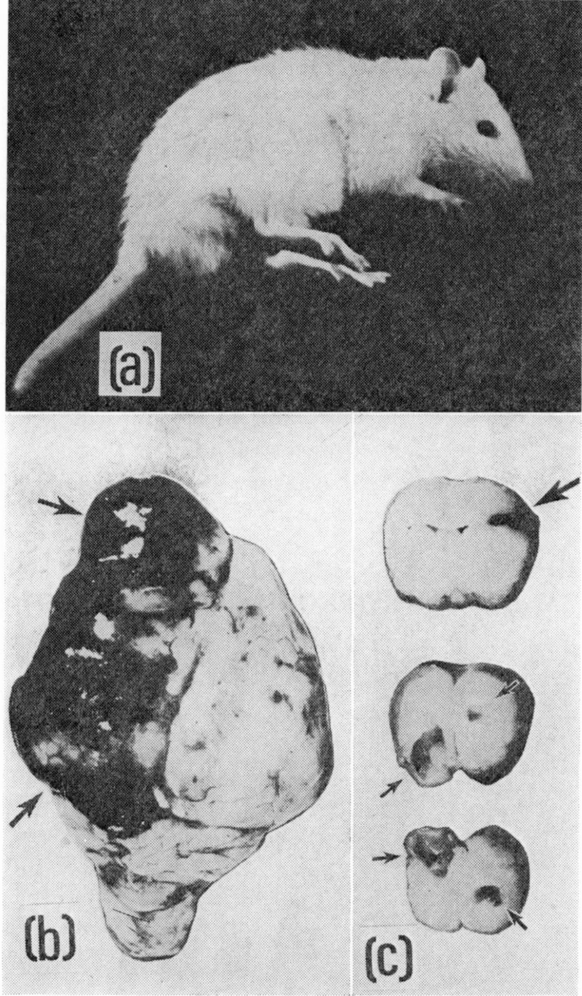

FIG. 3. (a) A 10-month-old stroke-prone SHR, with paralysis in the hind limbs after the attack of stroke. (b) Massive cerebral hemorrhage noted in an 8-month-old stroke-prone SHR. (c) Extensive softening at the basal ganglia noted in the coronal section of the brain of a 13-month-old stroke-prone SHR (small and large arrows indicate softening and hemorrhage, respectively).

the incidence of stroke in male F_1 and F_2 generations was 80 percent and 24 percent, respectively. On the other hand, the F_1 and F_2 generations obtained by the crosses between stroke-prone SHR and normotensive rats showed an intermediate average blood pressure between those of parent strains. Although no stroke was observed in the F_1 generation with moderate hypertension, stroke was observed in 7 percent of the F_2 segregants with severe hypertension. Although a conclusion is not possible at present, so far the inheritance of stroke seems to be closely related to the heredity of severe hypertension.

Not only the genetic factor, but also environmental factors, are involved in the development of stroke. For example, substrain A_3 had a higher incidence of stroke (47 percent) than substrain C (4 percent). Salt-loading increased the incidence in both substrains, 78 percent in A and 18 percent in C, respectively, but substrain differences in the incidence of stroke were observed even under the altered dietary conditions (Figure 4) (Okamoto, Yamori, Nosaka, Ooshima, and Hazama, 1973). This experiment clearly

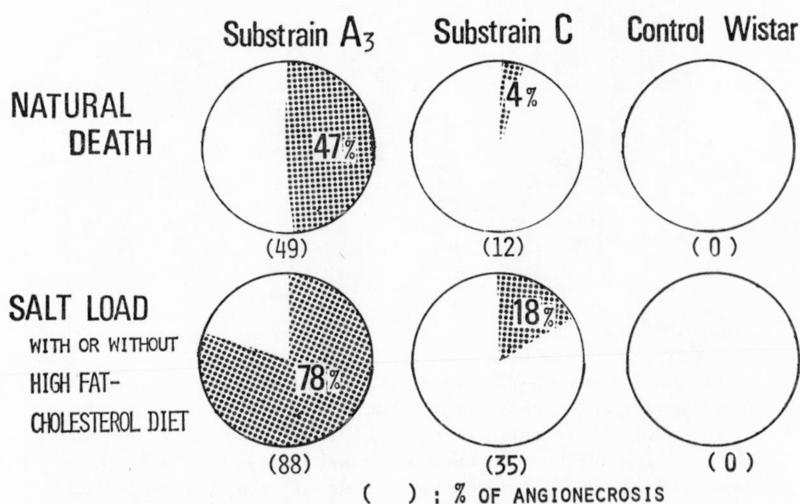

FIG. 4. Effect of salt-loading on the incidence of stroke in SHR-substrains with different predisposition to stroke. Numbers in parentheses are percentages of angionecrosis.

showed the importance of gene-environmental interaction for the development of stroke.

Pathogenesis of stroke. Our studies on the pathogenesis of stroke in these rats clarified the following systemic and local factors: The highly significant correlation between the incidence of stroke and the severity of hypertension or the speed of development of hypertension in various SHR substrains clearly indicated that the rapid development of hypertension over 200 mmHg was the important factor in stroke (Yamori, Nagaoka, and Okamoto, 1974). Other systemic factors are humoral factors such as renin, and possible alterations in the physicochemical characteristics of the arterial wall (Yamori and Sasagawa, 1974). Plasma renin concentration was increased in stroke-prone SHR over the age of six months which already had angionecrosis in the kidney or in the brain (Matsunaga, Yamamoto, Hara, Yamori, Ogino, and Okamoto, 1975). This finding indicates that renin is related to arterial lesions, either primarily or secondarily.

Our analysis of local factors in stroke indicated that the predilection sites of stroke in more than 1,200 stroke-prone SHR were the anteromedial and occipital cortex and basal ganglia, in contrast to the fact that the incidence of stroke in humans was highest in the basal ganglia. These predilection sites (the cortex and basal ganglia in rats and the basal ganglia in humans) had a common angioarchitectural characteristic: predilection sites of stroke, both in rats and in humans, were angiographically confirmed to be fed by the recurrent arteries branching from the parent artery (Yamori, Horie, Sato, Handa, and Fukase, 1975). Since recurrent branchings seem to be a common local factor in stroke, such branchings may be the base for hemodynamic derangement inducing the insufficiency of local blood supply. Our recent work actually proved that regional cerebral blood flow in the areas fed by recurrent arteries was decreased in a severe hypertensive state over 200 mmHg (Yamori, Horie, Sato, and Handa, 1976). A decrease in cerebral blood flow increases vascular permeability due to hypoxia and induces angionecrosis. Microangiographical and histopathological studies showed the formation of microaneurysms and hemorrhage due to the rupture of microaneurysms; at the site of cerebral softening, arteries were occluded with thrombosis formed at microaneurysms or the arterial wall with angionecrosis.

In summary, hypertension is the most important systemic factor in stroke; some other factors may be involved, either primarily or secondarily. Under the influence of a severe hypertensive state, local factors such as recurrent branchings seem to be the base for the decreased regional cerebral blood flow, which causes vascular damage due to hypoxia and finally increases vascular permeability or induces angionecrosis. Angionecrosis and thrombosis at the site of angionecrosis or microaneurysms are the basic common vascular lesions for both hemorrhage and softening. Therefore, stroke in these rats is the "angionecro-thrombogenic stroke" seen in hypertensive patients in Japan.

Prophylaxis of stroke. Although stroke is caused mainly by genetic factors related to severe hypertension, alteration of environmental factors against these mechanisms seems to be effective in preventing stroke. The most effective prophylaxis of stroke is obviously the control of severe hypertension. No stroke was observed in stroke-prone SHR treated with antihypertensive agents from the prehypertensive stage: their blood pressure was maintained at less than 210 mmHg, while stroke was observed in 80 percent of nontreated stroke-prone SHR (Yamori and Horie, 1975). In all these experiments, the litter from the same parents was divided into treated and non-treated groups, so that these two groups had similar genetic dispositions.

Epidemiological studies show that the incidence of stroke, both hemorrhage and infarction, is higher in males than in females. As a similar tendency was observed in stroke-prone SHR, we treated males with estrogen and females with androgen in order to observe the effect of altered hormonal conditions on stroke (Yamori, Sato, Horie, and Ohta, 1976). Estrogen treatment (estradiol; 40 μg/kg/week, i.m.) attenuated the development of hypertension in males. The treated males showed blood pressure similar to that in non-treated females. On the other hand, androgen treatment (testosterone; 5 mg/kg/week, i.m.) accelerated the development of hypertension in females. The treated females quickly developed severe hypertension similar to that of non-treated males. An androgen-treated female already showed signs of stroke, such as paralysis and urinary incontinence, at a young age, but an estrogen-treated male was apparently healthy and developed stroke later in the advanced stage. In conclusion, estrogen treatment in males decreased the incidence of stroke, while androgen treatment in females increased the incidence, and the results indicated the importance of humoral endocrine factors for the development of stroke.

Another epidemiological study showed a clear difference in the incidence of stroke in various countries; the incidence is very high in Japan in comparison with European countries and the U.S.A. As such environmental factors as nutrition may be related to the marked difference in the incidence of stroke, we have been observing the effect of various nutritional conditions on the incidence of stroke in the stroke-prone SHR. So far as we observed, a hypercholesterolemic diet dramatically decreased the incidence of stroke, and such a marked decrease in incidence seems to be related to the attenuation of severe hypertension in stroke-prone SHR fed on a hypercholesterolemic diet (Yamori, Sato, and Horie, 1976). The worst nutritional condition was a low-protein diet plus salt water, which clearly shortened the life span, augmented hypertension, and increased the incidence of stroke within a short period. On the other hand, a high-protein diet was confirmed to be very effective, and no stroke was observed in the stroke-prone SHR fed on a diet containing 50 percent protein. These experimental findings indicated that high-protein and high-fat diets decreased the incidence of stroke and suggest that a marked epidemiological difference in the incidence of stroke between Japan and western countries may be mainly due to nutritional conditions.

A New Model for Atherogenesis

The SHR is not only a good model for stroke research, but was recently confirmed to be a good model for atherogenesis research, although rats had been regarded as inadequate experimental animals for atherogenesis.

An SHR substrain fed on a hypercholesterolemic diet (consisting of 20 percent suet, 5 percent cholesterol, and 2 percent cholic acid) quickly developed hypercholesterolemia (500–800 mg/dl) within a week when salt water was given concomitantly (Yamori, 1974). They have been selected for greater hypercholesterolemic responses, and F_6 generations have been obtained. When fed on hypercholesterolemic diets, they developed ring-like fat deposits in mesenteric arteries within a week (Figure 5) and in cerebrobasal arteries within a few weeks. These fat deposits in cerebrobasal arteries were only observed in SHR and experimental hypertensive rats fed on hypercholesterolemic diets, and were never noted in normotensive rats. When SHR were fed on hypercholesterolemic diets plus salt water, fat depositions quickly developed in the mesenteric artery within a week. Furthermore, when hypertension was well controlled by antihypertensive agents, arterial fat deposition was greatly delayed in mesenteric arteries; only a few rings were noted after hypercholesterolemic diet feeding for nearly two months. Consequently, hypertension was shown to be an important factor in acute arterial fat deposition, the initial process of atherogenesis. Although such fat deposits were never noted in normotensive Wistar rats, some fat deposits were detected in the mesenteric arteries of SHR, even when their blood pressure was normalized with antihypertensive

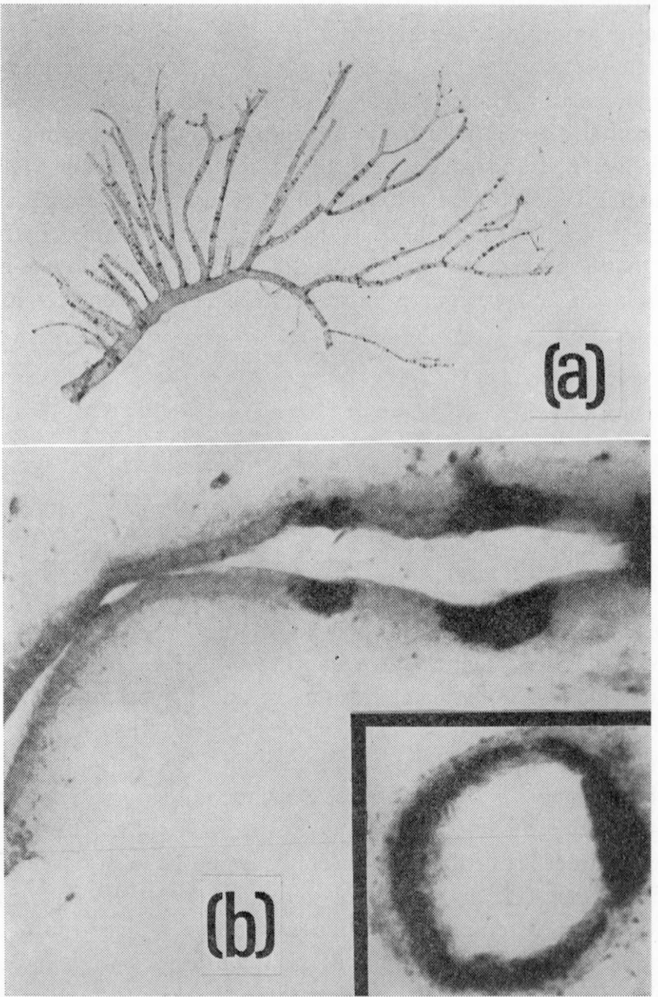

FIG. 5. Arterial fat deposition in SHR. (a) Ring-like fat deposits in the mesenteric artery of SHR fed on a high-fat-cholesterol diet. (b) Sudan stained histological section of the mesenteric artery.

agents. Consequently, hypertension and hypercholesterolemia, both of which are induced by gene and environmental interactions, are obviously important in arterial fat deposition. Moreover, genetic disposition, probably related to vascular permeability, may be involved in arterial fat deposition, the initiation process of atherogenesis.

In conclusion, most common vascular lesions are classified into hypertensive and lipidemic angiopathy, according to the findings on SHR. The former are hypertensive vascular lesions causing stroke and nephrosclerosis, and the latter are athero- or arteriosclerosis. Under gene and environmental interactions, three main factors—hypertension, lipidemia, and vascular permeability—seem to be the basis for these two types of vascular lesions. Our experimental data up to the present suggest that hypertension plus increased vascular permeability cause angionecrosis, which is the basis for stroke and malignant nephrosclerosis. On the other hand, lipidemia with increased vascular permeability causes atherosclerosis in systemic arteries such as mesenteric arteries, and lipidemia plus hypertension is the basis for atherogenesis also in cerebral arteries.

Our studies on spontaneous hypertension showed the importance of genetic predisposition and its interaction with environmental factors in the pathogenesis of hypertension, stroke, and atherogenesis. The control of gene-environmental interaction is expected to prevent these common diseases in man in the near future; our experiments have shown successful examples of such prophylaxis in animal models.

REFERENCES

Aoki, K., Yamori, Y., Ooshima, A., and Okamoto, K. 1972. Effects of high or low sodium intake in spontaneously hypertensive rats. *Japan. Circ. J.* **36**: 539–545.

Dahl, L. K., Heine, M., and Tassinari, L. 1962. Effects of chronic excess salt ingestion. Evidence that genetic factors play an important role in susceptibility to experimental hypertension. *J. Exp. Med.* **115**: 1173–1190.

Folkow, B., Hallbäck, M., Lundgren, Y., Sivertsson, R. ,and Weiss, L. 1973. Importance of adaptive changes in vascular design for establishment of primary hypertension, studied in man and in spontaneously hypertensive rats. *Cir. Res.* **32**, **33**, Suppl. 1: 2–16.

Matsunaga, M., Yamamoto, J., Hara, A., Yamori, Y., Ogino, K., and Okamoto, K. 1975. Plasma renin and hypertensive vascular complications; an observation in the stroke-prone spontaneously hypertensive rat. *Jap. Circ. J.* **39**: 1305–1311.

Okamoto, K. 1969. Spontaneous hypertension in rats. (*International review of experimental pathology*, ed. by Richter, G. W., and Epstein, M. A., Academic Press, New York and London) No. 7, p. 227–270.

Okamoto, K., and Aoki, K. 1963. Development of a strain of spontaneously hypertensive rats. *Jap. Circ. J.* **27**: 282–293.

Okamoto, K., Yamori, Y., and Nagaoka, A. 1974. Establishment of the stroke-prone SHR. *Circ. Res.* **34**, **35**, Suppl. 1: 143–153.

Okamoto, K., Yamori, Y., Nosaka, S., Ooshima, A., and Hazama, F. 1973. Studies on hypertension in spontaneously hypertensive rats. *Clin. Sci. Mol. Med.* **45**: 11s–14s.

Smirk, F. H., and Hall, W. H. 1958. Inherited hypertension in rats. *Nature* **182**: 727–728.

Tanase, H., Suzuki, Y., Ooshima, A., Yamori, Y., and Okamoto, K. 1970. Genetic analysis of blood pressure in spontaneously hypertensive rats. *Jap. Circ. J.* **34**: 1197–1212.

Yamori, Y. 1974. Contribution of cardiovascular factors to the development of hypertension in spontaneously hypertensive rats. *Jap. Heart J.* **15**: 194–196.

Yamori, Y. 1974. Metabolic pathology of vasculatures in hypertension and vascular lesions in spontaneously hypertensive rats. *Trans. Soc. Path. Jap.* **63**: 226–227.

Yamori, Y. 1975. Interaction of neural and non-neural factors in the pathogenesis of spontaneous hypertension. (*The nervous system in arterial hypertension*, ed. by Julius, S., and Esler, M., C. C. Thomas, Springfield, Ill., U.S.A.) p. 17–43.

Yamori, Y., and Horie, R. 1975. Experimental studies on the pathogenesis and prophylaxis of stroke in stroke-prone spontaneously hypertensive rats (SHR). (2) Prophylactic effect of moderate control of blood pressure on stroke. *Jap. Circ. J.* **39**: 607–611.

Yamori, Y., Horie, R., Sato, M., and Handa, H. 1976. Pathogenetic similarity of stroke in stroke-prone spontaneously hypertensive rats and humans. *Stroke* **7**: 46–53.

Yamori, Y., Horie, R., Sato, M., and Handa, H. 1976. Regional cerebral blood flow in stroke-prone SHR. *Jap. Heart J.* **17**: 384–386.

Yamori, Y., Matsumoto, M., Yamabe, H., and Okamoto, K. 1969. Augmentation of spontaneous hypertension by chronic stress in rats. *Jap. Circ. J.* **33**: 399–409.

Yamori, Y., Nagaoka, A., and Okamoto, K. 1974. Importance of genetic factors in hypertensive cerebrovascular lesions; an evidence obtained by successive selective breeding of stroke-prone and -resistant SHR. *Jap. Circ. J.* **38**: 1095.

Yamori, Y., and Sasagawa, S. 1975. Physico-morphological characteristics of aorta in stroke-prone and -resistant spontaneously hypertensive rats. *Jap. Heart J.* **15**: 296–298.

Yamori, Y., Sato, M., and Horie, R. 1976. Blood pressure and vascular lesions in SHR fed on a high-fat-cholesterol diet. *Jap. Heart J.* **17**: 396–398.

Yamori, Y., Sato, M., Horie, R., and Ohta, K. 1976. Prophylactic trials for stroke in stroke-prone SHR: Effect of Sex Hormones. *Jap. Heart J.* **17**: 410–412.

Embryogenesis of Human Limb Malformations Compared with Those in Animals

Mineo Yasuda

Introduction

Many reports have been published on pathogenesis of congenital malformations in experimental animals. In contrast, we have only scanty information on this matter in man. The knowledge of abnormal morphogenesis in human embryos is invaluable for extrapolation to man of teratological findings in experimental animals. A large collection of normal and abnormal human embryos at the Human Embryo Center for Teratology, Faculty of Medicine, Kyoto University, has provided us with unique opportunities to study the early processes involved in the formation of certain congenital malformations in man.

Limb malformations are relatively common in Japanese. Baba *et al.* (1967) reported that limb malformations were found in newborns at a rate of 2.7 per 1,000, and that they accounted for about one-third of gross external malformations. The purpose of this presentation is to describe the morphogenesis of certain limb malformations in man and in experimental animals, and to discuss possible applications of the obtained information to the prevention of congenital malformations.

Human Embryonic Materials

A large number of human embryos—so far more than 37,000—have been collected at the Human Embryo Center for Teratology, Faculty of Medicine, Kyoto University. Details of the collection have been described elsewhere (Nishimura *et al.*, 1966, 1968). They were obtained from mostly healthy women whose pregnancies had been terminated. These embryos were fixed

Department of Perinatology, Institute for Developmental Research, Aichi Prefectural Colony, Aichi, Japan.

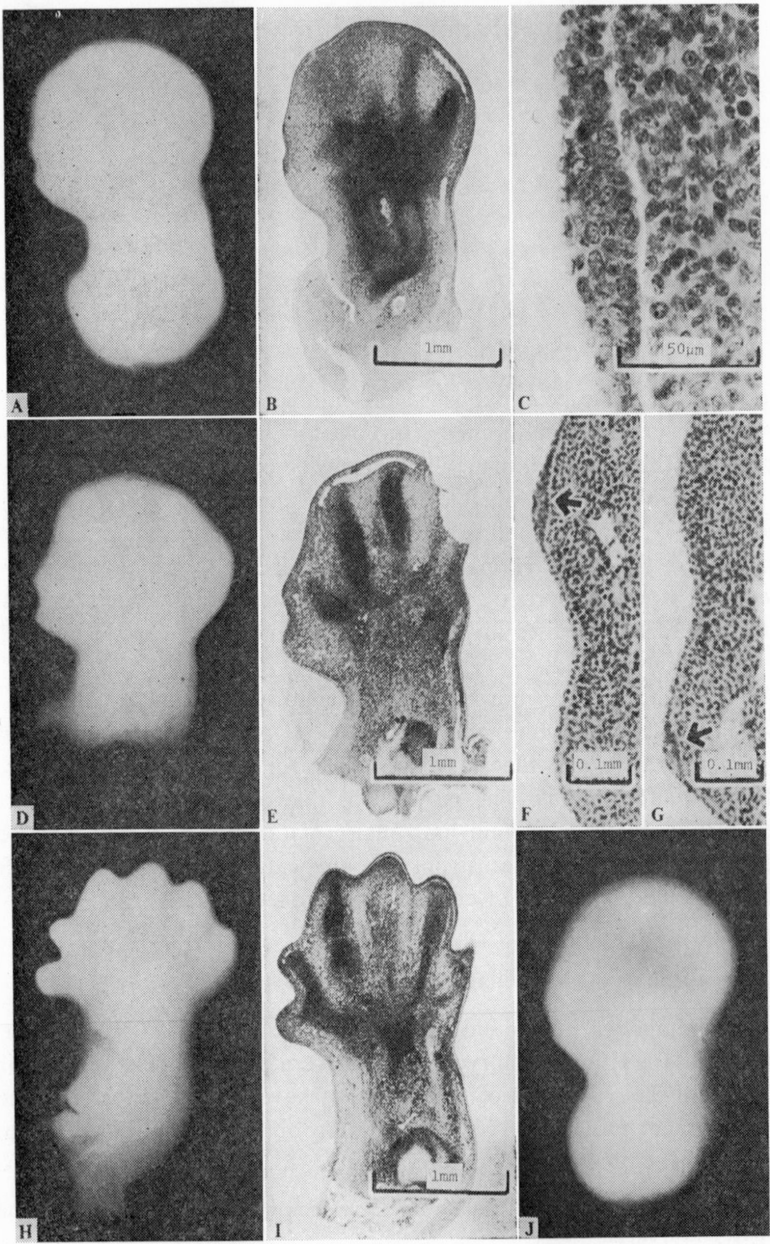
A
B
1mm
C
50μm
D
E
1mm
F
0.1mm
G
0.1mm
H
I
1mm
J

in Bouin's fluid, staged according to the criteria described by Streeter (1942, 1945, 1948, 1951) and modified by O'Rahilly (1972), and examined for possible external malformations under a binocular dissecting microscope. Specimens without signs of intrauterine death were used for the study of pathogenesis of congenital malformations.

Embryogenesis of Limb Deformities

Preaxial polydactyly. Preaxial polydactyly of the hand (radial polydactyly) was one of the common types of malformations found in Japanese embryos (Nishimura, 1970). Its pathogenesis was described by Yasuda (1975a). A human hand plate first exhibits digital rays at stage 17. At this stage an early indication of preaxial polydactyly can be detected with certainty (Figure 1A). Histological observations revealed the following morphological features in early pathogenesis of preaxial polydactyly: (1) abnormal extension and a delayed involution of the apical ectodermal ridge (AER) on the preaxial border of the hand plate in stages 17 and 18 (Figures 1B, C, and E-G); (2) precocious development of an interdigital notch between the duplicated thumbs in stages 17 and 18 (Figures 1A and D); and (3) bifurcation of the distal part of the first digital ray in stage 19 (Figure 1I). These findings suggested that small tubercles occasionally found on the preaxial border of the hand plate in stage 16 (Figure 1J) might be a precursor of polydactyly. Histological observations and a survey of the prevalence rates of those tubercles in embryos at stages 16, 17, and 18 indicated a strong tendency for the preaxial tubercle to develop into polydactyly (Yasuda and Nakamura, 1972). Abnormal morphogenesis of preaxial polydactyly in human embryos is diagrammatically summarized in Figure 3.

FIG. 1. Pathogenesis of preaxial polydactyly.

A. Dorsal view of a right hand plate with preaxial polydactyly at stage 17.
B. A section of the hand plate shown in A. Note epidermal thickenings at the preaxial margin.
C. Higher magnification of the epidermal thickening.
D. Dorsal view of a right hand plate with preaxial polydactyly at stage 18.
E. A section of the hand plate shown in D.
F. and G. Epidermal thickenings at the tip of the two protrusions.
H. Dorsal view of a right hand plate with preaxial polydactyly at stage 19.
I. A section of the hand plate shown in H. The first finger ray is bifurcated. There is no conspicuous epidermal thickening.
J. Dorsal view of a right hand plate with preaxial tubercles at stage 16.

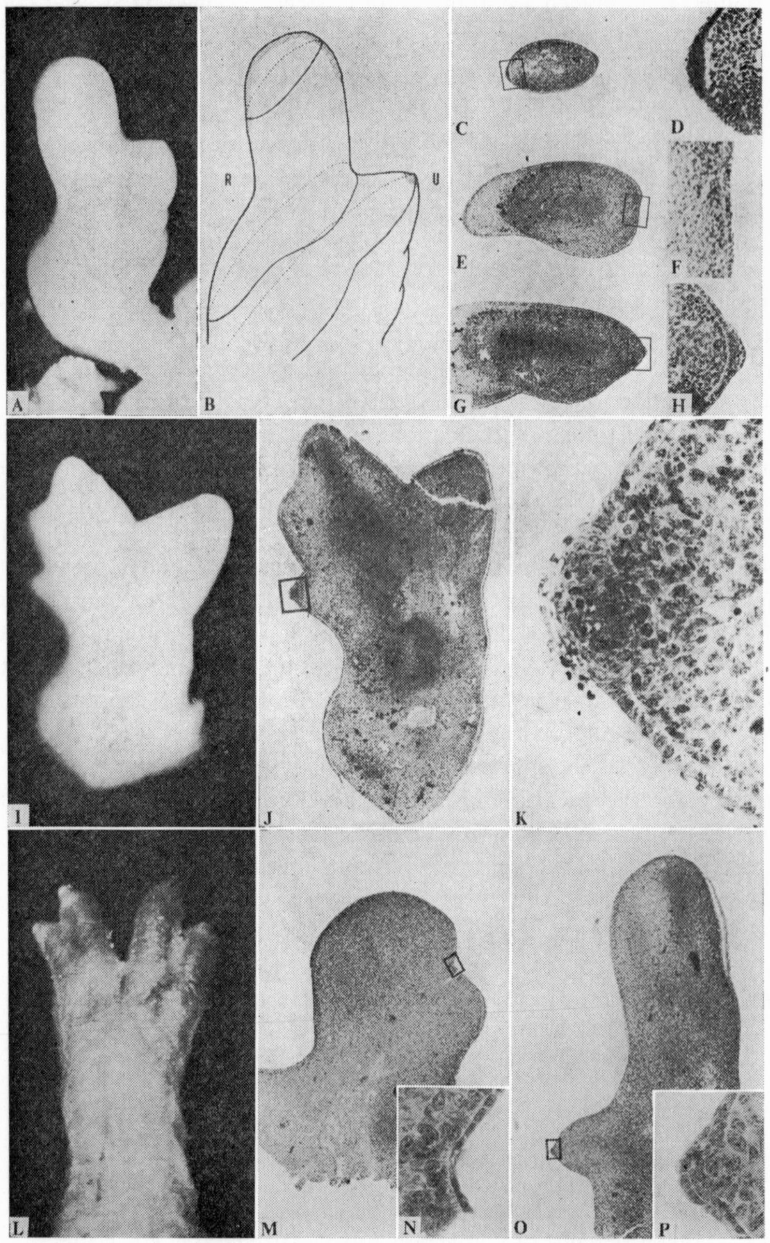
A
B
R
U
C
D
E
F
G
H
I
J
K
L
M
N
O
P

Abnormalities of the AER have been described in the development of polydactyly in experimental animals. Zwilling and Hansborough (1956) found a preaxial enlargement associated with preaxial extension of the AER in the limb buds of four-day "duplicate" chick embryos as the first indication of the duplicate condition. Kameyama *et al.* (1974) detected preaxial extension of the AER and its delayed involution in the foot plate of mouse embryos treated on day 10 with 5-fluorouracil as the early changes in the formation of preaxial polydactyly. These findings suggest that a disorder of the interaction between limb ectoderm and mesoderm is the pathogenetic event leading to polydactyly.

Cleft hand. A different type of abnormal development of the AER was found in the process of cleft formation in the human hand plate (Yasuda, 1971a, 1975b). Observations of serial sections of hand plates with clefts in stage 16 revealed that the rim along the defect lacked the AER (Figures 2B–H), which is present continuously along the entire apical rim of a normal hand plate in stage 16. A stage 18 hand with cleft showed precocious formation of the interdigital notches and delayed involution of the AER

FIG. 2. Pathogenesis of cleft hand.

A. Dorsal view of a right upper limb bud with cleft at stage 16.

B. A diagram showing the direction of sectioning and the level of sections appearing in C–G. Stippled areas indicate the AER. R=radial; U=ulnar.

C. and D. A section through the distal part of the limb bud, and higher magnification of epidermis. The AER is seen on the radial and ulnar sides.

E. and F. A section through the cleft, and higher magnification of epidermis. The AER is absent.

G. and H. A section through the tip of the ulnar portion. A small area is covered with the AER.

I. Dorsal view of a right hand plate with cleft at stage 18.

J. A section of the hand plate shown in I.

K. Higher magnification of the tip of the first finger. A conspicuous epidermal thickening is present.

L. Dorsal view of a right forepaw of a term fetus of the "meromelia" mouse.

M and N. A section of a forelimb bud of an 11-day embryo of the "meromelia" mouse, and higher magnification of thin epidermis covering the cleft.

O. and P. A section of a forelimb bud of a 12-day embryo of the "meromelia" mouse, and higher magnification of thickened epidermis covering the tip of the radial portion.

(Figures 2I–K). Observations of the development of a cleft hand-like deformity in a mutant strain of mice are in progress. This mutant was recently discovered by Prof. K. Kondo and his associates of the Department of Animal Breeding, Faculty of Agriculture, Nagoya University, and tentatively designated as "meromelia," since animals which are homozygous for the recessive mutant gene (*mem/mem*) develop various types of limb deformities ranging from polydactyly to severe hemimelia. Homozygous meromelia C57BL/6 mice occasionally exhibit an interdigital cleft in the fore- or hindpaw (Figure 2L). Histological examination of hand plates with cleft of *mem/mem* embryos revealed interruption of the AER at the site of cleft and delayed involution of the AER (Figures 2M–P). Pathogenesis of cleft hand is diagrammatically summarized in Figure 3.

Hemimelia. Early morphological features of hemimelia were also studied in human embryos at stages 13 (just after formation of the upper limb bud) through 16 (just before formation of the finger rays) (Yasuda, 1975c). One specimen at stage 13 showed an increase of pyknotic cells in the limb bud

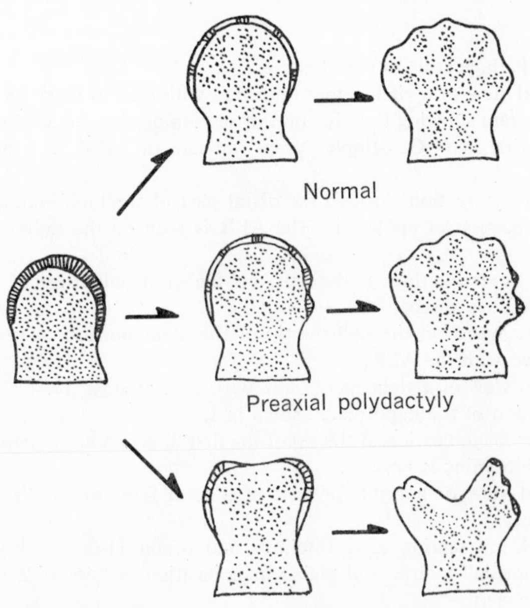

FIG. 3. The AER, finger rays, and interdigital notches in the formation of normal, polydactylous, and cleft hands.

mesenchyme (Figures 4B and C), whereas no conspicuous cellular abnormality was noted in the specimens at stages 14 and later (Figures 4F and G). No aberration in the microscopic structure of the AER was detected, although in the hemimelic limb the size of the AER was reduced (Figures 4F and G).

Massive mesenchymal necrosis in the limb bud was found to lead to limb reduction deformities in mouse embryos treated with an excessive amount of vitamin A on day 10 of gestation (Yamawaki *et al.*, 1974). In this animal model, however, the developmental stage of the limb bud with massive cell death was around the time of foot plate formation and was more advanced than stage 13 of human embryos.

Usefulness of Information on Embryogenesis of Human Malformations

Evaluation of animal models. The examples given in the previous section clearly show that there are some common features between man and animal models in the embryogenesis of limb malformations. Extrapolation to man of data obtained in these animal models may be warranted on the basis of these similarities. Diseases in animal models, however, may differ from those in humans in various ways. A study without critical evaluation of the animal model employed may be useless for prevention of human congenital malformations. The knowledge of embryogenesis of human malformations provides indispensable feedback for the evaluation of animal models and for the development of better animal models.

Early diagnosis of malformations in embryos. Recognition of early pathogenetic features of malformations enables us to diagnose malformations precisely in small human embryos. For example, it is possible to diagnose preaxial polydactyly by detection of preaxial tubercles of the AER at stage 16 when no digital rays are recognizable. Diagnosis of malformations in embryos has practical applications, because abortuses may be utilized as materials for genetic counselling (Poland and Lowry, 1974) and for monitoring of new environmental teratogens (Miller and Poland, 1971).

Creation of hypothesis explaining phenotypic variations. Understanding of an abnormal morphogenetic process may lead to a hypothesis explaining variations in a certain morphological features. For example, there are variations in preaxial polydactyly ranging from broad thumb to complete duplication of the first metacarpus. These may be due to variations in the extension of the AER on the preaxial border of the hand plate. It might

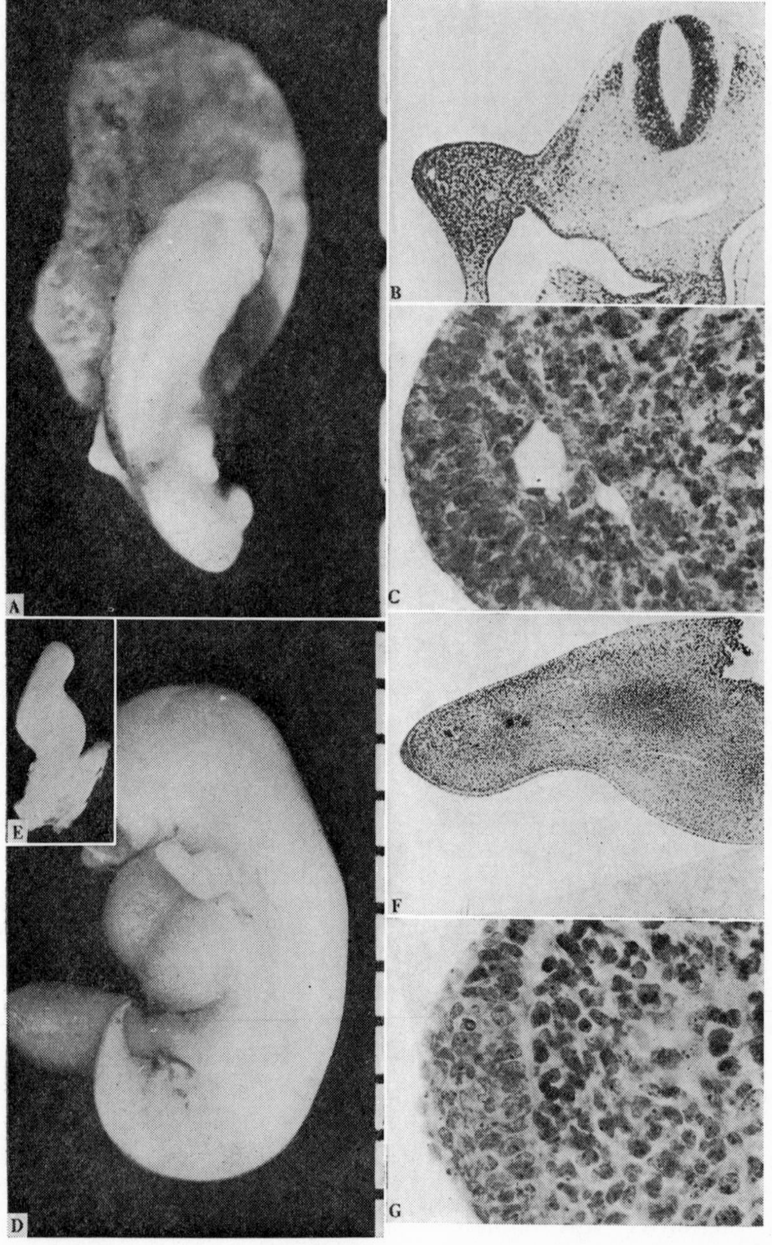
A
B
C
D
E
F
G

be justified to apply the quasi-continuity theory to the genesis of preaxial polydactyly, because Ohkura (1956) suggested a gene with low penetrance and environmental factors as causes of polydactyly among Japanese. It is possible to assume that the liability for polydactyly may be determined by the degree of extension of the AER on the preaxial border of the hand plate at a certain developmental stage (Figure 5). If some morphological

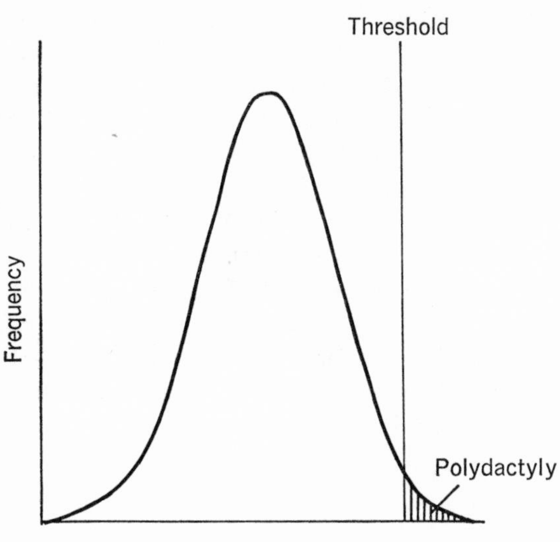

FIG. 5. Explanation of the genesis of preaxial polydactyly by the quasi-continuity theory. An embryo with the AER extended on the preaxial border over the threshold level at a certain developmental stage is considered to become polydactylous.

FIG. 4. Pathogenesis of hemimelia.

A. Dorsal view of a stage 13 embryo with hypoplastic upper limb buds.
B. A cross section of the embryo shown in A through the upper limb bud.
C. Higher magnification of the upper limb bud. Note numerous pyknotic nuclei in limb mesenchyme in contrast to intact epidermis.
D. View of the left side of a stage 15 embryo with hemimelic upper limbs.
E. Dorsal view of the hemimelic left upper limb.
F. A section of the limb bud shown in E.
G. Higher magnification of a distal part of the limb bud. Note the intact AER and mesenchymal cells.

features of a completed hand, such as the relative size of the thumb and the dermatoglyphic pattern, reflect the degree of extension of the AER at a certain embryonic stage, these features may be used to measure the individual's liability to reproduce a child with polydactyly.

Evolution of a better taxonomic scheme of dysmorphogenesis. Epidemiological and genetic studies of human congenital malformations require a systematic classification of anomalies. The present state of classification and nomenclature of malformations, especially of malformation syndromes, is far from systematic. To diminish the taxonomic chaos, Herrmann and Opitz (1974) proposed several fundamental concepts, including "developmental field complex (DFC)," and Pinsky (1975) recommended the classification of syndromes on the basis of phenotypic resemblances (communities). Descriptions of pathogenesis will serve in the evolution of a better taxonomic scheme by providing a basis to explain DFCs and the formal genesis of communities of malformation syndromes. For example, a difference in pathogenesis between preaxial and postaxial polydactyly was detected by Yasuda (1971b). No extension of the AER was noted in the formation of postaxial polydactyly. Limb malformations may be divided into those with AER abnormalities and those without, although the significance of this kind of categorization remains to be studied.

Conclusions

There are two major methods of studying gene-environmental interaction in the causation of congenital malformations: one is genetic epidemiology in man, and the other is experimental teratology in animal models. Comparative descriptions of embryogenesis of malformations in man and experimental animals serve as a bridge between these two methods.

REFERENCES

Baba, K., Takeya, H., Okada, T., Nakamura, J., and Otsuka, S. 1967. Twenty-years review of congenital abnormalities born in a hospital in Tokyo. *Nihon Univ. Med. J.* **26**: 420–429.

Herrmann, J., and Opitz, J. M. 1974. Naming and nomenclature of syndromes. *Birth Defects Orig. Art. Ser.* X/7: 69–86.

Kameyama, Y., Hoshino, K., and Hayashi, I. 1974. Morphogenesis of 5-fluorouracil induced polydactylism in mice. Epithelial-mesenchymal interactions in the formation of polydactylism. *Ann. Rep. Res. Inst. Environ. Med. Nagoya Univ.* **21**: 59–66.

Miller, J. R., and Poland, B. J. 1971. Monitoring of human embryonic and fetal wastage. *Monitoring, birth defects and environment*, pp. 65–81, Academic Press, New York, U. S. A.; London, U. K.

Nishimura, H., Takano, K., Tanimura, T., Yasuda, M., and Uchida, T. 1966. High incidence of several malformations in the early human embryos as compared with infants. *Biol. Neonate.* **10**: 93–107.

Nishimura, H., Takano, K., Tanimura, T., and Yasuda, M. 1968. Normal and abnormal development of human embryos: First report of the analysis of 1,213 intact embryos. *Teratology* **1**: 281–290.

Nishimura, H. 1970. Incidence of malformations in abortions. *In* Fraser, F. C., and McKusick (Eds.), *Congenital malformations*, pp. 275–283, Excerpta Medica, Amsterdam, the Netherlands.

Ohkura, K. 1956. Clinical genetics of polydactylism. *Jap. J. Hum. Genet.* **1**: 11–23.

O'Rahilly, R. 1972. Guide to the staging of human embryos. *Anat. Anz.* **130**: 556–570.

Pinsky, L. 1975. The community of human malformation syndromes that shares ectodermal dysplasia and deformities of the hands and feet. *Teratology* **11**: 227–242.

Poland, B. J., and Lowry, R. B. 1974. The use of spontaneous abortuses and stillbirths in genetic counseling. *Am. J. Obstet. Gynecol.* **118**: 322–326.

Streeter, G. L. 1942. Developmental horizons in human embryos: Description of age group XI, 13 to 20 somites, and age group XII, 21 to 29 somites. *Contrib. Embryol.* **30**: 211–245.

Streeter, G. L. 1945. Developmental horizons in human embryos: Description of age group XIII, embryos about 4 or 5 millimeters long, and age group XIV, period of indentation of the lens vesicle. *Contrib. Embryol.* **31**: 27–63.

Streeter, G. L. 1948. Developmental horizons in human embryos: Description of age group XV, XVI, XVII, and XVIII, being the third issue of a survey of the Carnegie Collection. *Contrib. Embryol.* **32**: 133–203.

Streeter, G. L. 1951. Developmental horizons in human embryos. Description of age groups XIX, XX, XXI, XXII, and XXIII, being the fifth issue of a survey of the Carnegie Collection. *Contrib. Embryol.* **34**: 165–196.

Yamawaki, H., Nakamura, H., Fujisawa, H., and Yasuda, M. 1974. Effects of maternal hypervitaminosis A upon developing mouse limb buds. I. Light microscopic investigation. *Cong. Anom.* **14**: 13–22.

Yasuda, M. 1971a. Early morphogenesis of cleft hand in human embryos. *Acta Anat. Nippon.* **46**: 19–20 (Abst.)

Yasuda, M. 1971b. Early morphogenesis of postaxial polydactyly in human embryos. *Proc. Cong. Anom. Res. Ass. Jap.* **11**: 36. (Abst.)

Yasuda, M. 1975a. Pathogenesis of preaxial polydactyly of the hand in human embryos. *J. Embryol. Exp. Morph.* **33**: 745–756.

Yasuda, M. 1975b. Abnormal apical ectodermal ridge and cleft hand formation in human embryos of stages 16–17. *In* Yamada, E. (Ed.), *Proceedings Tenth Int. Cong. Anat.*, p. 125. Science Council of Japan, Tokyo, Japan.

Yasuda, M. 1975c. Pathogenesis of reduction deformity of the upper limb in human embryos. *Teratology* **12**: 218. (Abst.)

Yasuda, M., and Nakamura, H. 1972. Early pathogenesis of polydactyly: Pre- or postaxial tubercle on the hand plate of human embryos at the stage of digital ray formation. *Teratology* **6**: 125. (Abst.)

Zwilling, E., and Hansborough, L. A. 1956. Interaction between limb bud ectoderm and mesoderm in the chick embryo. III. Experiments with polydactylous limbs. *J. Exp. Zool.* **132**: 219–239.

Animal Models of Common Diseases: Comparative Developmental Pathology of Central Nervous System Malformations

Yoshiro Kameyama

The application of teratological findings from laboratory animals to the pathogenesis of central nervous system malformations in the human presents various difficulties. The great phylogenetic difference in cerebral organization between man and animals and the diversity of causal factors of malformations constitute serious obstacles to comparative studies. Species difference in the length of fetal period is another important factor which brings about marked discrepancies in final states of malformations (Kameyama, 1971). However, the morphogenetic investigation of central nervous system malformations in laboratory animals, if these originated from abnormalities in the early developmental stage, will present useful information for human malformations, since the developing brain and spinal cord during organogenesis and early histogenesis are similar in different species of mammals.

In order to analyze complex problems involving genetic and environmental factors which interact during the intrauterine period, it is necessary first to understand the teratological characteristics of the developing nervous system and the sequential processes leading to the abnormal phenotypes.

In this presentation, I would like first to cover the teratological characteristics of the central nervous system which have been recognized in experimental teratology.

Teratological Characteristics of the Central Nervous System

The central nervous system malformations in laboratory animals which are comparable to those in humans can be divided into two groups according to the developmental stage at which initial changes occur: organogenetic malformations and histogenetic malformations.

Research Institute of Environmental Medicine, Nagoya University, Nagoya, Japan.

TABLE 1. Organogenesis of cerebrum.

Man (W)	Mouse (Days)	Organogenesis	Developmental disorder	Organogenetic malformations
2	6–7	Neural plate		Exencephaly
			Dysraphism	Encephalomeningocele
3	7–8	Neural tube		Meningocele
3–4	8	Prosencephalon		
			Failure to divide	Holoprosencephaly
4	9	Telencephalon		

In the first critical period of organogenesis, the neural tube closes at the cephalic and caudal portions. In the second, the single prosencephalic vesicle divides into two telencephalic vesicles. Some failure in the process during the first period brings about various types of dysraphic malformations such as exencephaly, myeloschisis, encephalocele, myelocele, meningocele, and spina bifida. A failure in the second period causes holoprosencephaly (Table 1).

The experimentally-induced organogenetic malformations are strictly stage-specific in their manifestations, since both closure of the neural tube and division of the prosencephalic vesicle occur within a short time—less than one day in rats and mice. The undifferentiated neural tissue during organogenesis is highly sensitive to teratogenic factors and is easily subject to degenerative changes. Nevertheless, it also has an active regenerative capacity in the event of tissue damage (Table 3). Consequently, the manifestation of organogenetic malformations is characterized as "all or none" at birth.

The histogenesis of the brain proceeds with proliferation of the undifferentiated neural cells in the periventricular matrix, migration of the post-mitotic differentiating neural cells toward the outer zone of the brain mantle, formation of the cortical plate, formation of the laminar structure of the cortex, and cytodifferentiation of neuroblasts in the cortex. Any disturbance of these processes produces histogenetic malformations such as microcephaly, dysgenetic hydrocephaly, absent corpus callosum, heterotopic cortical gray matter, disorganized cortical structure, and underdevelopment of the cortical neurons (Table 2). Therefore, the experimentally-induced histogenetic malformations of the brain mantle are not strictly stage-spacific in their manifestations, and their sensitive periods are much longer than those of organogenetic ones. The sensitivity of the differentiat-

TABLE 2. Histogenesis of brain mantle.

Man (W)	Mouse (Days)	Histogenesis	Developmental disorder	Histogenetic malformations
6	11	Start of cell migration	Disturbance of proliferation, migration	Dysgenetic hydrocephaly Microcephaly Absence of corpus callosum
8–9	13	Primordial cortex		Heterotopic gray matter
20	17	Termination of production of cortical neurons		Disorganized cortical architecture
20∼	Birth∼	Laminar architecture of cortex		
24∼	Postnatal 1–2 W	Differentiation of neuroblast of cortex		
7 M		Major cerebral gyri		
9 M	1–2 W	Myelination		

TABLE 3. Experimentally induced malformations of CNS.

	Organogenetic malformation	Histogenetic malformation
Sensitive period	Period of organogenesis	Fetal, neonatal periods
Stage-specificity	⧺	+∼−
Cellular vulnerability	⧺	+
Repair activity	⧺	+∼−
Histological aberration	+	⧺
Primary disturbance of cell differentiation and growth	+∼−	⧺

ing neural tissue to teratogenic agents during histogenesis lowers markedly with fetal age, but so does the capacity for repair. As a result, histological abnormalities such as deficit of neurons and aberrant neural structure can hardly be repaired (Table 3). This may be one of the main reasons why histogenetic malformations are more prevalent than those of the organogenetic type.

The morphological features of histogenetic malformations are apt to be altered from the original states of maldevelopment by degenerative changes, due to disturbance of blood circulation, hemorrhage, and failure of the secretion-absorption mechanism of the cerebrospinal fluid—all of which occur as secondary changes of histological aberration of the developing neural tissue.

These findings in laboratory animals suggest that developmental disorders of the brain mantle are probably one of the important causal factors of cerebral lesions which manifest themselves in the late fetal or postnatal periods. From this point of view, I will review and discuss the developmental pathology of congenital hydrocephaly, of both genetic and environmental origins, in laboratory animals.

Developmental Pathology of Congenital Hydrocephaly in Laboratory Animals

The morphological investigation of congenital hydrocephaly provides useful models for understanding the human congenital hydrocephaly, since this malformation manifests itself in almost all mammalian species, and the final morphological features are similar among different species of mammals. It has been difficult, in many cases, to point out a single formal origin of congenital hydrocephaly after it became evident.

The congenital hydrocephalias in laboratory animals which are comparable to those in humans can be classified into five groups according to the site of the main pathological change detected in the earlier fetal period: Dandy-Walker-type malformation of the fourth ventricle; developmental disturbance of the meninges and subarachnoid space; stenosis and obstruction of the Sylvian aqueduct; Arnold-Chiari-type hindbrain malformation; and histogenetic disorders of the brain mantle.

Dandy-Walker-type hydrocephaly. Regarded as belonging to the Dandy-Walker type are two genetic hydrocephalias in mice, hydrocephalus-1 (*hy*−1) and dreher (*dr*), and a garactoflavin-induced hydrocephaly in mice. According to the reports on these three hydrocephalias by Bonnevie (1943), Deol (1964), and Kalter (1963), the common characteristics were cystic enlargement of the roof of the fourth ventricle and cerebellar hypoplasia. The enlargement of the fourth ventricle was already detectable on day 12 to 14 of gestation as a bulging state of the epithelial roof. The cerebellar hypoplasia was marked in the median part and was regarded as a consequence of the enlargement.

The morphological features of these three hydrocephalias closely resemble the human Dandy-Walker malformation described by Benda (1954) and D'Agostino *et al.* (1963). The findings in mice suggest that human Dandy-Walker malformations can originate from histological abnormalities of the roof of the fourth ventricle, and can be caused by either genetic or environmental factors in the early gestation period.

Developmental disturbance of the meninges and subarachnoid space. The developmental disturbance of the meninges and subarachnoid space has been regarded as the cause of two genetic hydrocephalias in mice: hydrocephalus-3 (*hy*-3) and congenital hydrocephalus (*ch*).

Berry (1961) reported that hydrocephalus-3 (*hy*-3) showed a cloudy degeneration of the meninges which appeared first around the fourth ventricle in the neonatal period and spread over the whole cerebral surface. He concluded that this cloudy degeneration was probably a cause of blockage of the cerebrospinal circulation.

The mutant gene *ch* of congenital hydrocephalus has been known to bring about pleiotropically various malformations in the mesodermal structure, such as skeletal and urogenital systems (Grüneberg, 1953). Green (1970) and Grüneberg *et al.* (1974) reported that a bulging of the roof of the fourth ventricle and an underdevelopment of the subarachnoid space appeared on day 13 to 15 of gestation. They postulated that the primary cause of this hydrocephaly was a failure of cerebrospinal fluid to flow into the subarachnoid space due to a defect of this space.

These pathological changes have not been described in human hydrocephaly, but the findings in the two mutant mice suggest that not only morphological but also functional disorders of subarachnoid space may be causal factors of human congenital hydrocephaly.

Stenosis and obstruction of the Sylvian aqueduct. The stenosis and obstruction of the aqueduct have been found frequently in genetic and teratogen-induced hydrocephalias of laboratory animals (Kalter, 1968; Warkany, 1971). But it is difficult to determine whether or not an obstruction or the stenosis is really the initial cause leading to an accumulation of cerebrospinal fluid, except when "forking" or blind end is observed. Because stenosis and obstruction can easily be brought about in immature brains by sequential changes in the process of hydrocephalic formation such as intra- or periventricular hemorrhages, ependymal ablation, and mechanical pressure from the cerebrum. Emery (1974) pointed out that the aqueduct can be obliterated simply by the compression of the occipital poles on the brain stem before it is fully myelinated.

Arnold-Chiari-type malformation of the hindbrain. The hindbrain malformation of the Arnold-Chiari type has been produced experimentally in rat fetus by maternal administration of trypan-blue. According to reports by Gunberg (1956), Warkany *et al.* (1958), and Vickers (1961), the caudal dislocation of the hindbrain and cerebellum into the cervical spinal canal in the rat fetus was remarkably similar in morphology to the human Arnold-Chiari malformation. This hindbrain malformation was frequently accompanied by myeloschisis in the late fetal offspring, but not by apparent hydrocephaly, although reduction or obliteration of the subarachnoid cisternas could be occasionally found. None of the animals with myeloschisis had hydrocephaly. It was also noticed that only one hindbrain malformation, myeloschisis or hydrocephaly, was manifest in a litter.

The causal relationships among the above three malformations have not yet been established in the experimentally-induced Arnold-Chiari-type malformation.

Histogenetic disorders of the brain mantle. Dysgenetic hydrocephaly is the condition in which the ventricular system remains in the large-vesicle stage due to a developmental arrest of the brain mantle, and has been regarded as a different morbid entity from true hydrocephaly in the human. However, postnatal delayed manifestation of hydrocephaly has been observed often in laboratory animals involved with the dysgenetic one in the fetal and neonatal periods. Postnatal hydrocephaly was also found in mice which had been involved with microcephaly in the perinatal period.

Chamberlain (1970) reported that mice with dysgenetic hydrocephaly induced in the fetal period by 6-aminonicotinamide revealed hydrocephaly after birth. He reported that this final anomaly appeared to be caused by an obstruction of the cerebrospinal fluid circulation at or beyond the fourth ventricle.

Shimada *et al.* (1974) reported that hydrocephaly occurred in infant mice in which dysgenetic hydrocephaly had been induced in the neonatal period by prenatal treatment with cytosine arabinoside. They suggested that this late manifestation of hydrocephaly might be attributed to a failure of the production-absorption mechanism of cerebrospinal fluid resulting from an extensive defect of the ependymal layer of the ventricular system, and also to an aqueductal stenosis by ependymal ablation and gliosis.

The author and his co-workers observed the postnatal changes of X-ray-induced microcephaly in sequence in mice which had been exposed to 200R in the fetal period, and also found a postnatal manifestation of hydrocephaly (Kameyama *et al.*, 1972). In the group irradiated on day 12 and after day 14 of gestation, the microcephalic state remained unchanged. In the group treated on day 13, the lateral ventricles of the microcephalic

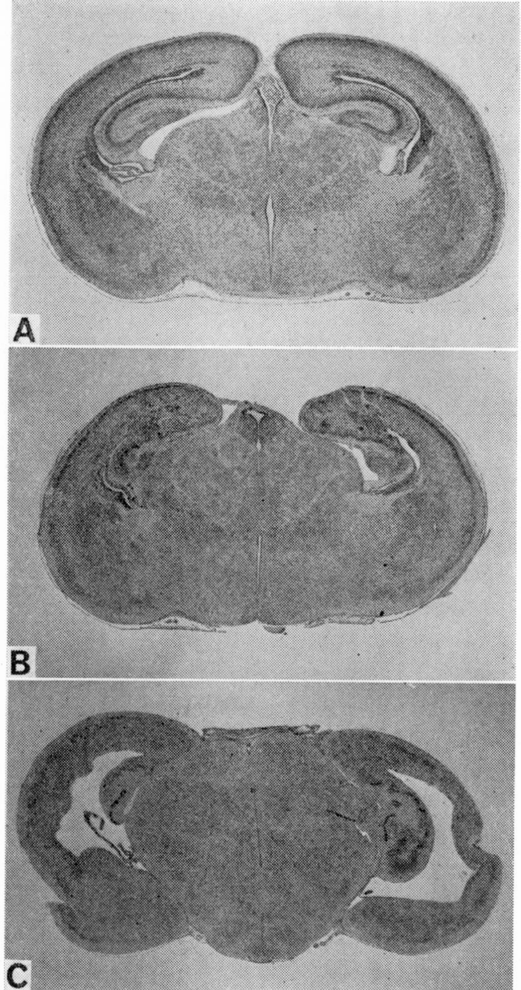

FIG. 1. Coronal sections of the brains of CF #1 mice (gallocyanine stain).

A. Normal brain of newborn mouse in the untreated control group.

B. Microcephaly of newborn mouse in the group treated with 200R of x-ray on day 13 of gestation. The development of the dorsal neocortex and hippocampus is severely disturbed.

C. Hydrocephaly of 14-day-old mouse in the same group as B. The brain mantle is reduced in thickness and the lateral ventricles are markedly enlarged (Kameyama *et al.*, 1972).

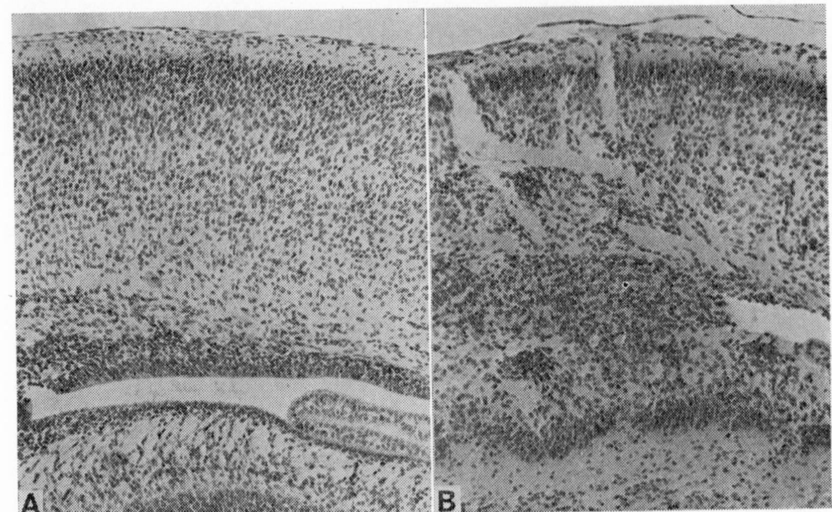

FIG. 2

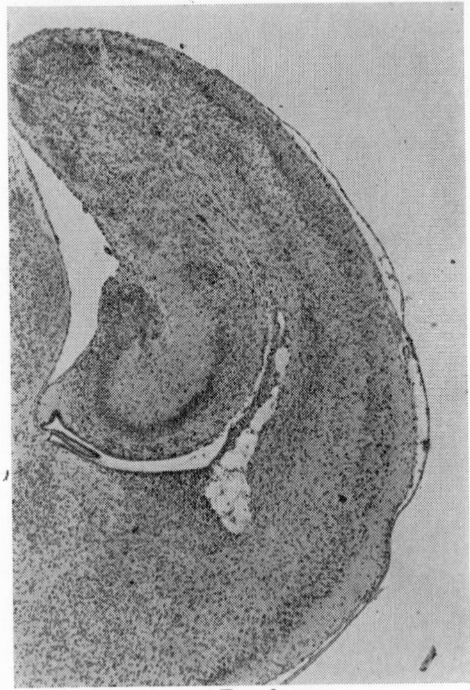

FIG. 3

mice started to enlarge one to two weeks after birth, and hydrocephaly became intensive progressively with advance of age (Figure 1).

It was noticed that postnatal hydrocephaly occurred in brains involved with marked histological aberration of the brain mantle (Figure 2). Prior to the manifestation of hydrocephaly, venous congestion, periventricular hemorrhages, and subsequent tissue defects were evident in the brain mantle in the neonatal period (Figure 3). In order to know whether the pathogenesis of circulatory disturbance occurred postnatally, the brains were examined in vascular specimens with india ink. Abnormal vascular pattern and poor vascular network of the brain mantle were demonstrated to exist in the microcephalic brains with disorganized cortical structure (Figure 4) (Kameyama *et al.*, 1972).

These results suggested that prenatal abnormal vascular formation in the brain mantle with aberrant histological structure caused cerebral venous congestion with hemorrhages postnatally, and that these vascular disorders might bring about tissue damage and a failure in the dynamics of the cerebrospinal fluid (Figure 5).

Recently, causal relationships between fetal circulatory disorders in the brain and congenital communicating hydrocephaly have drawn the attention of neuropathologists (Granholm *et al.*, 1963; Lourie *et al.*, 1965; Towbin, 1968). Histogenetic disorders of the fetal brain may be one of the important causal factors not only of human congenital hydrocephaly, but also of cerebral lesions which take place during the perinatal period and result in cerebral palsies and mental deficiencies after birth.

FIG. 2. Dorsal parts of the neocortices of newborn mice in the coronal sections cutting through the optic chiasma (H. E. stain).

A. Normal neocortex in the untreated control group.

B. Malformed neocortex in the group irradiated with 200R of x-ray on day 13 of gestation. Aberration of cortical structure and heterotopia are evident (Kameyama *et al.*, 1972).

FIG. 3. Coronal section of the brain of 7-day-old mouse in the group irradiated with 200R on day 13 of gestation (gallocyanine stain). Tissue defect following hemorrhage is seen in the subependymal white matter at the lateral edge of the lateral ventiricle (Kameyama *et al.* 1972).

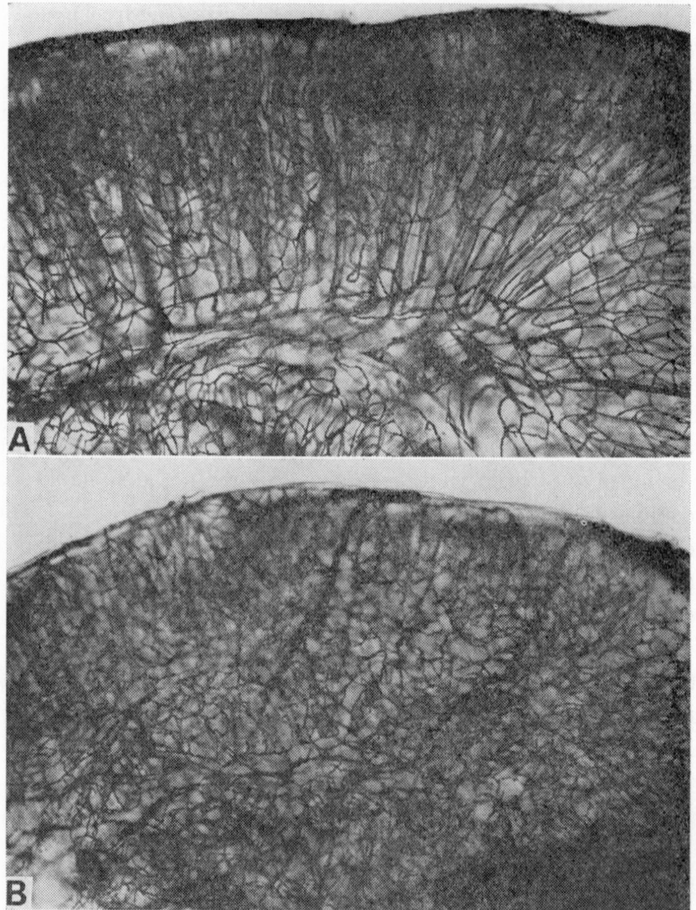

FIG. 4. Vascular specimens (with india ink) of the dorsal neocortices of 14-day-old mice.

A. Normal vascular pattern in the untreated control group. The long perforating cortico-medullary vessels traverse the cortex perpendicularly to the surface and are arranged regularly. The short perforating vessels form an arcade-like network in the cortex.

B. Abormal vascular pattern in the group irradiated with 200R on day 13 of gestation. The vascular pattern is markedly deranged and the perforating cortico-medullary veins are strongly dilated (Kameyama *et al.*, 1972).

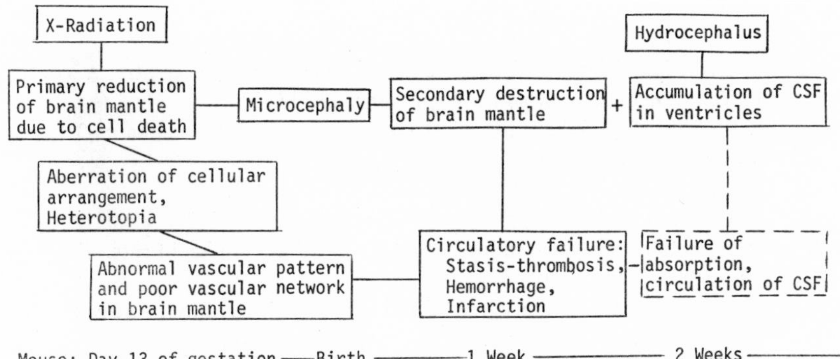

FIG. 5. Morphological sequences from X-ray-induced tissue damage of the fetal brain to postnatal hydrocephaly in mice (Kameyama *et al.*, 1972).

SUMMARY

The pathogenesis of central nervous system malformations is very difficult to assess by postnatal observation alone, since the morphological expressions can be altered by sequential changes such as failure of neuro-mesenchymal interactions, tissue degeneration, and vascular abnormalities, and original developmental disorders are occasionally masked by predominant secondary destructive tissue damages.

In this presentation, teratological characteristics of the central nervous system were introduced and the developmental pathology of congenital hydrocephaly in laboratory animals was reviewed and discussed.

Developmental pathological studies on central nervous system malformations, of both genetic and environmental origins, in laboratory animals have served to elucidate the processes of maldevelopment. Embryological studies by classical methods of observation provide useful models for understanding the course from the initial morphological change to the complex abnormal phenotype, and will contribute to the problem of combinant effects of the genetic and evnironmental processes taking place in the intrauterine period.

Acknowledgement

The author wishes to thank Dr. Ujihiro Murakami, Director of the Institute for Developmental Research, Aichi Prefectural Colony, Aichi, for his valuable advice on this presentation.

REFERENCES

Benda, C. E. 1954. The Dandy-Walker syndrome or so-called atresia of the foramen Magendie. *J. Neuropath. Exp. Neur.* **13**: 14–29.

Berry, R. J. 1961. The inheritance and pathogenesis of hydrocephalus-3 in the mouse. *J. Pathol. Bact.* **81**: 157–167.

Bonnevie, K. 1943. Cited from Kalter, 1968, pp. 191–203.

Chamberlain, J. G. 1970. Early neurovascular abnormalities underlying 6-aminonicotinamide (6-AN)-induced congenital hydrocephalus in rats. *Teratology* **3**: 377–388.

D'Agostino, A. N., Kernohan, J. W., and Brown, J. R. 1963. The Dandy-Walker syndrome. *J. Neuropath. Exp. Neur.* **22**: 450–470.

Deol, M. S. 1964. The origin of the abnormalities of the inner ear in Dreher mice. *J. Embryol. Exp. Morphol.* **12**: 727–733.

Emery, J. L. 1974. Deformity of the aqueduct of Sylvius in children with hydrocephalus and myelomeningocele. *Dev. Med. Child Neurol.* **16**: Suppl. No. 32, 40–48.

Granholm, L., and Radberg, C. 1963. Congenital communicating hydrocephalus. *J. Neurosurg.* **20**: 338–343.

Green, M. C. 1970. The developmental effects of congenital hydrocephalus (*ch*) in the mouse. *Dev. Biol.* **23**: 585–608.

Grüneberg, H. 1953. Genetic studies on the skeleton of the mouse. VII. Congenital hydrocephalus. *J. Genet.* **51**: 327–358.

Grüneberg, H., and Wickramaratne, G. A. 1974. A re-examination of two skeletal mutants of the mouse, vestigial-tail (*vt*) and congenital hydrocephalus (*ch*). *J. Embryol. Exp. Morphol.* **31**: 207–222.

Gunberg, D. L. 1956. Spina bifida and the Arnold-Chiari malformation in the progeny of trypan-blue injected rats. *Anat. Rec.* **126**: 343–367.

Kalter, H. 1963. Experimental mammalian teratogenesis, a study of galactoflavin-induced hydrocephalus in mice. *J. Morphol.* **112**: 303–317.

Kalter, H. 1968. *Teratology of the central nervous system.* pp. 21–184. Univ. of Chicago Press, Chicago, U.S.A.

Kameyama, Y. 1971. Comparative developmental pathology of congenital malformations of the central nervous system. *Brain and Development* **3**: 450–459.

Kameyama, Y., and Hoshino, K. 1972. Postnatal manifestation of hydrocephalus in mice caused by prenatal X-radiation. *Cong. Anom.* **12**: 1–9.

Kameyama, Y., Hayashi, Y., and Hoshino, K. 1972. Abnormal vascularity in the brain mantle with X-ray induced microcephaly in mice. *Cong. Anom.* **12**: 147–156.

Lourie, H., and Berne, A. S. 1965. A contribution on the etiology and pathogenesis of congenital communicating hydrocephalus. *Neurology* **15**: 815–822.

Shimada, T., Kasubuchi, Y., Wakaizumi, S., and Nakamura, T. 1974. Congenital hydrocephalus in mice following transplacental administration of drugs. *In*

Kawabuchi, J. (Ed.), *Spina bifida and congenital hydrocephalus*, pp. 22–25. Neuronsha, Tokyo, Japan.

Twobin, A. 1968. Cerebral intraventricular hemorrhage and subependymal infarction in the fetus and premature newborn. *Am. J. Pathol.* **52**: 121–139.

Vickers, T. H. 1961. Die experimentelle Erzeugung der Arnold-Chiari Missbildung durch Trypan-blau. *Beitr. Pathol. Anat.* **124**: 295–310.

Warkany, J., Wilson, J. G., and Geiger, J. F. 1958. Myeloschisis and myelomeningocele produced experimentally in the rat. *J. Comp. Neurol.* **109**: 35–64.

Warkany, J. 1971. *Congenital malformations, notes and comments*, pp. 217–231. Year Book Medical Pub., Chicago, U.S.A.

DISCUSSION 1

Gunn Rat as a Model for Unconjugated Hyperbilirubinemia in Infancy

Kazuo Baba

I am going to discuss the usefulness of the Gunn rat as an animal model for human neonatal jaundice and other unconjugated hyperbilirubinemia in infancy.

In 1964, Dr. Arias kindly gave us four pairs of homozygous Gunn rats. Though the attempt to get some offspring from these pairs in our own laboratory did not succeed, Dr. Suzuki and other members of Sankyo Central Research Laboratories succeeded in propagating jaundiced rats by crossing Gunn rats with Wister-Imamichi rats.

They confirmed that the best way for maintenance and propagation of jaundiced rats is to mate a homozygous male with heterozygous female. Although the pure bred strain has not been established, successive back-crosses have been continued in order to introduce the jaundice gene into Wister-Imamichi strain. Most of jaundiced rats, which are used in this country under the name of Gunn rat, may have been derived from this hybrid.

It has long been confirmed that the basic defect of homozygous Gunn rats is hepatic glucuronyl transferase deficiency, and the defect is transmitted as an autosomal recessive trait. Jaundice is noticed by 6 hours of age, and persists throughout life. Bilirubin in the serum gives an indirect van den Bergh reaction, and the level varies from 5 to 20 mg/dl. About 70 percent of homozygous animals develop neurological signs caused by kernicterus in second or third week after birth. Postmortem examinations of the brain revealed kernicterus similar to that of human subjects (Table 1).

Comparing the Gunn rat with human diseases, characteristic features of Gunn rat are identical to those of Crigler-Najjar syndrome. Basic defect of these abnormalities is hepatic glucuronyl transferase deficiency, which is responsible for severe unconjugated hyperbilirubinemia and kernicterus.

Gilbert's disease, neonatal jaundice, and erythroblastosis are in part similar to Gunn rats, because all of these illness are characterized by re-

Nihon University School of Medicine, Tokyo, Japan.

duced glucuronyl transferase activity and elevated serum unconjugated bilirubin (Table 2).

Though Crigler-Najjar syndrome is an extremely rare disease, the Gunn rat has served as an excellent model to study many problems relating to bilirubin metabolism and kernicterus (Table 3).

TABLE 1. Biologic Features of Gunn Rats.

Enzyme Defect	:	UDPGT deficiency
Inheritance	:	Autosomal recessive
Symptoms	:	Jaundice Neurol. Sign
Blood Chemistry	:	Unconj. Hyperbilirubinemia (5–20 mg/dl)
Pathol. Findings	:	Kernicterus (65–75%)
Mortality	:	20–80%

TABLE 2. Comparison with Human Diseases.

	Hemolysis	UDPGT Activity	Unconjugated Bilirubin	Kernicterus
Gunn Rat	0	0	↑↑	⧻
Crigler-Najjar S.	0	0	↑↑	⧻
Gilbert's D.	0	↓	↑	0
Neonat. Jaundice	↑	↓	↑	+
Erythroblastosis	↑↑	↓	↑↑	++

TABLE 3. Usefulness of Gunn Rats.

Useful Characteristics	Relevant Subjects of the Study
UDP-GT Deficiency	Effect of Phenobarbital Toxicity of Drugs
Hyperbilirubinemia	Effect of Phototherapy
Kernicterus	Kernicterogenic Factors Toxicity of Bilirubin

DISCUSSION 2

Breeding of Disease Model Mice

Kyoji Kondo

The genetic improvement of mice as a laboratory animal means to prepare suitable mice for each biomedical experiment or to prepare suitable disease models. However, the meaning of "suitable" is an important and complicated problem. The disease is also a diverse and complicated phenomenon. But the syndrome is manifested based on the two factors, namely genetical and environmental ones.

It is common knowledge that inbred strains are ideal tools for studying the nature of biomedical character, including disease. By using inbred mice or rats, we can analyze the disease at a definite genetical level. So at the first step, we may conclude that the breeding of inbred strains is an important means of genetical improvement. But each inbred strain has its own specific character based on its gene constitution. For this reason, the next step is to match or adjust the specific character of the inbred strain to each research or "disease model."

The specificity in genetic character of the inbred strain is mainly derived from the following two factors: 1) selection through sib-inbreeding, 2) original source or gene pool from which inbred strains are bred. The selection method is a well known method for "good matching." The SHR rat strain bred by Okamoto and Aoki is a good example for the disease model of "hypertension," based on the selection method.

However, the sib-inbreeding over 20 generations according to a definite selection schedule requires several years and the procedure might not always be successful. The breeding of disease model should be always performed according to dual schedules: special genetic character and good reproductive performance. Frequently the dual selection schedules give rise to difficulties. However sib-inbreeding based on only the reproductive performance is not so difficult and inbred strains bred according to the schedule of selection are different in their genetical characters because of two factors: differences in original source and random genetic drift. Therefore, we propose a second method of good matching: the aptitude test method.

Department of Animal Breeding, Nagoya University, Nagoya, Japan.

The procedure for the aptitude test method is as follows. When some specific disease model is required in research, a suitable test or tests for finding the specific character are carried out among maintained inbred strains. Usually we can find the strain differences in the results of testing, and suitable strains can be chosen from the results.

In Japan, we have many different origins of mice from which inbred strains are bred. The origins can be classified into five original foundations. The first one is *Mus musculus molossinus*, Japanese wild mouse. The second group consists of fancy mice. The third group is descendants of laboratory mice imported from Europe with the advent of modern medicine. The fourth group is native dealer's stock, supposed to be mongrels of several origins. The fifth group came from the United State as improved laboratory strains after the second world war. The fifth group is not a single population, but can be classified into several different family trees. The abundant resources for breeding of inbred strains can be prepared from these various groups and the crosses among them. About 50 inbred strains of mice have been bred from these sources and further breedings are now in progress.

As we have many different kinds of inbred strains, as noted above, the aptitude test method should be successful. For example, useful strains for research on diabetes mellitus: KK, KSB, and AY, have been found by the tests "urine sugar and blood sugar content" by Nishimura. Ino and Yoshikawa also found several strains by alloxan treatment test. Actually, there are merits and demerits in both methods as shown in Table 1.

TABLE 1. Comparison between two methods.

	Selection method	Aptitude test method
Start	Require "polymorphic original gene pool"	Require "many established inbred strains, differing in gene constitution"
Procedure	Selection and inbreeding	Decision of aptitude test and testing the provided inbred strains
Time required	Several years	Possible in a set time
Results	Usually, one or two useful inbred strains	Several inbred strains differing in characters
Remarks	Through the procedure, genetical meaning of the required character may become clear	Genetic meaning of the difference remains unknown. Hopeless in the low reproductive trait, because inbred strains are selected for good reproduction.

The genetic disease model not only is based on the specific inbred strains, but also depends on the mutant gene. For example, diabetic mutant genes — yellow lethal (Ay), adipose (ad), diabetes (db) and obese (ob) — have been found and used as useful mutants. The combination of these two, characteristics of inbred strains and major mutant genes, is an interesting method of breeding, and congenic inbred strains, KK-Ay, KSB-Ay, etc., are important animal models.

The next problem is how to pick up the major gene itself. The major gene of disease model is a useful tool for analyzing the gene action, and we find the mutant gene in our usual observation. However, the discovery of a useful mutant gene is only by chance and the direction of mutation is unknown. It is possible to increase the rate of mutation by X-ray or other mutagens, but at present it is impossible for us to gain the suitable mutant gene.

DISCUSSION 3

Monophasic and Diphasic Morphogenesis of Some Malformed Organs in Mammalian Development

Ujihiro Murakami

When conducting teratological experiments employing mammals, stage factors (stage specificity) are one of the best known principles in morphogenesis.

I have been working in the field of comparative developmental pathology, i.e., experimental teratology, for many years, and I have come to realize fully the importance of stage factors. I would like to show some examples of a phenomenon I have come across; in particular, what I call a diphasic elevation of incidence in the manifestation of malformations from the viewpoint of morphogenesis.

Malformations Caused by Extrinsic Factors Showing A Monophasic Elevation of Incidence

The first example is the manifestation of arhinencephalias in the mouse exposed to X-irradiation from 150R to 300R on day 7 to 12 of pregnancy. The day of pregnancy had been determined by examination of females with vaginal plugs to be in day zero of pregnancy in the morning after mating. Then, I found many cases of arhinencephalias, though they displayed a single spectrum in their manifestations. In this case, the peak of incidence manifesting the pattern was observed in those exposed on day 8 and showed a monophasic elevation of incidence.

The second monophasic example is microcephalias. L. B. Russell, (1952) called this pattern a "vaulted cranium." Histopathologically, these turned out to be hydromicrocephalias.

The third monophasic example is cleft palate produced by hypervitaminosis A. The incidence of cleft palate was higher (70 percent) in middle pregnancy.

Institute for Developmental Research, Aichi Prefectural Colony, Kasugai, Japan.

Malformations Caused by Extrinsic Factors Showing a Diphasic Elevation of Incidence

The first example is manifestation of malformation of the eye ranging from microphthalmia to anophthalmia.

The CF♯1 and ddN mice were subjected to X-irradiation of 200R or 300R from day 7 to 12 of pregnancy. In the ddN mice, elevation of manifestation of the above malformations were seen in the groups treated on days 8 and 12, while in the CF♯1 mice, a higher incidence of these eye malformations was found only in the group exposed on day 7.

The second example is manifestation of hydrocephalia. The incidence of manifestation of the pattern of malformation was observed to increase in two experimental groups, i.e., the first elevation was presented in those exposed on day 9 and the second elevation was shown in those treated on day 11.

The third example is manifestation of cleft palate. L. B. Russell, and W. L. Russell, (1954) showed that there was a diphasic elevation of incidence following X-irradiation. I confirmed the finding, but the first peak I observed was not high enough. Giroud (1965), on the other hand, showed a much more marked result.

The fourth example is a little complicated and needs a detailed explanation; readers may refer to the original (Murakami *et al.*, 1963).

Discussion

In some malformations of certain organ systems, there were observed two phasic elevations of incidence of malformations, according to the agent employed. These findings suggest that there may exist two kinds of morphogenesis which produce the same malformation.

Incidence of one group of malformations indicates one peak, in such cases as arhinencephalia, hydromicrocephalia, a group with cleft palate (probably the primary cleft palate) etc. But some other malformations such as hydrocephalia, hypoplastic malformations of the eye, another group with cleft palate (probably the secondary cleft palate), and malformations of the vertebra, indicated a diphasic elevation of incidence, especially in the ddN mice.

The first peak of incidence may represent a very indirect effect, i.e., the influences on the inductory system, ancestral cells of the prospective organs, or the primordium just prior to its formation. The second peak may represent a direct effect upon the primordium of some organs themselves. Such diphasic peaks were observed in the sensitive period of development.

The first manifestation of indirect effect is subtle. Generally, such an indirect effect may result in suppression of the organ primordium just prior to its formation.

Concerning the direct effect, the first direct damage to the organ primordium was well defined. A good example is the progress of the radiation injury and repair in the eye-cup, or the morphogenesis in ectrodactylia.

IV NEW APPROACHES TO COMMON DISEASES

Program for the Analysis of Empiric Risk Data of Common Diseases

Akio Kudô

Introduction

Empiric risks to unborn children have recently been paid increasing attention in connection with genetic counselling (cf. Herndon, 1962). The classical formulas of risk for sibs are being modified or improved (Freire-Maia, 1973). This notion seems to have originated well before the time when sophisticated mathematical statistics, including statistical inference based on exact sampling, were available. It seems that everybody can agree that in order to determine empiric risk, we need a rather large body of data. When we have the notion of empiric risk in mind, we are not contemplating a situation where the law of simple Mendelian inheritance can be applied. Thus the methods for analyzing the empiric risk data are in the realm of analysis of frequency data.

In 1974, a survey on empiric risk data was organized by Dr. Furusho of Kagoshima University. Our survey includes nearly 50 diseases, and nearly 20 medical doctors are collecting data. The data resources are: (1) case reports already published, (2) hospital records from more than 50 locations, and (3) mail inquiries already conducted. Thus it has a rather experimental feature, in the sense that we are trying to organize data which have already been collected but are still scattered all over the country.

The survey had not been completed for any of the diseases as of January 1976; thus this is a preliminary report. I will discuss, first, the survey and its problems; second, some aspects of computor algorithms, on which Dr. Koichi P. Ito and I have been, for some years, concentrating our efforts; and, third, comparisons between the logit and the exponit models.

Department of Mathematics, Kyushu University, Fukuoka, Japan.

Survey and Related Problems

Because of the financial restrictions particularly caused by rapidly increasing wages, we had to abandon the idea of establishing a headquarters, where some number of clerical workers could be continually engaged in scrutinizing and coding. The doctors in charge are asked to supply the data after coding the information on the data sheets, so that they can be ready for punching and verifying. After a brief scrutiny, the cards are punched and printed, and then sent back to the doctors for examination. This method of performing initial steps of data collection may cause some confusion and/or difficulty.

For instance, the names of diseases are coded in two-digit numbers. A careless mistake may well distort the data. This error will be amplified if data collected in a particular hospital are consistently coded erroneously; such an error will never be corrected until the particular doctor who transmitted the codes detects the mistake. This kind of difficulty is also caused by the fact that data resources are scattered and that the original data are most probably kept confidential.

Take another example: our calender year is not four digits. 1976 is the 51st year of Showa, and, in our particular convention, it is to be coded 351. The age of onset of a disease sometimes cannot calculated by simple substraction of the year of birth from the year of onset. I feel that these difficulties are particularly associated with Japanese culture, where Chinese characters are widely used.

One of the benefits of studies on the Japanese population is that we have the family registration system, which furnishes such things as solid confirmations of consanguinity. Doctors are accustomed to getting information on pedigree related to patients. In our survey, the format is so designed that not only sibs of a proband but also remote relatives such as great-grandparents, cousins of parents, etc. (25 different types), can be coded.

Thses features have convinced me that before the analysis can be successfully completed, we will have to go back to the original data. As a result, I am contemplating a research proposal related to computer science and information systems. It calls for the cooperation of medical doctors, statisticians, and computer experts. One of the facets of this proposal is "cost-benefit analyses of the use of optical mark cards." In our language,

Chinese characters play an inevitable role; the use of optical mark cards will reduce the cost and eliminate the errors to a great extent. Everyone has his own opinion about how it will benefit us, but no systematic study has yet been made.

Another facet of the proposal is methodology on storage and retrieval of data involving pedigrees. In contemplating this, I have drawn on a previous paper on a method of calculating the inbreeding coefficient (Kudô, 1962) and its computerized version, which has not been published, and the work of Yasuda and Maruyama (1970) and the papers cited therein.

Some explanation might be needed of the term "information system." What I mean by this is analogous to MEDLARS and MEDLINE, where 0.3–0.4 million articles are classified and indexed in a year. Chemical Abstract Service is still bigger; it processes about 0.4–0.5 million articles in a year. These are successfully computerized data storage systems in the United States. In the field of mathematics, computerized information service has not been so successful, but there are the tapes of the Index of Mathematical Papers, a quarterly index journal containing 0.03–0.04 million articles each year.

A giant information service, such as MEDLARS, is said to be too big for research workers. In order to circumvent such difficulties, there is a recent development: a researcher's file. This is a software system for strorage and retrieval of information on scientific documents selected, classified, and indexed by the individual's own method (Arikawa, 1975; Arikawa and Kitagawa, 1975).

In our proposal, the materials to be stored in a file are taken from hospitals. A proband and related documents (including pedigree) correspond to a paper and its author. The name of the hospital and an index, such as a serial number, correspond to a journal name and its volume and number. Then what would correspond to the key words? This is one of the main questions to be investigated in our proposal. Before the technical aspects of computer use are discussed, there are such basic questions to be explored.

Program for the Analysis of Empiric Risk Data

The data on empiric risk now being collected are not yet made available, so demonstrations are using the data from a consanguinity study already published (Tanaka, 1973; Yamaguchi *et al.*, 1970).

In cooperation with Dr. Koichi P. Ito, I am undertaking extensive reanalyses of these data. The data from both the empiric risk and the consanguinity study are frequency data, and the algorithms and the logic in this reanalysis are believed to be very useful in the analysis of empiric risk data. One of the facets of our efforts is developing an algorithm for instructing a computer to perform a wide variety of analyses at the same time so that the programming load on research workers can be removed. In this process, we ought to get a large number of printouts, and the next issue is how to interpret the outcomes. Readers are referred to Ito and Kudô, 1975; Ito and Kudô, 1976; Kudô and Ito, 1975.

In the study of consanguinity effects, we tried three models of occurrence probability:

Probability of:	Occurrence	Non-occurrence
	P	$1-P$
LINEAR	Y	$1-Y$
EXPONIT	$1-e^{-Y}$	e^{-Y}
LOGIT	$e^Y/1+e^Y$	$1/1+e^Y$

where Y is a function of variables ($=(X_1, X_2, \ldots)$) explaining probability of occurrence or non-occurrence such as $Y=a_1X_1+a_2X_2+\ldots$. In the above equation $a_0, a_1, a_2, \ldots$ are coefficients to independent variables $X_0, X_1, X_2 \ldots$. If $X_0=1$, $X_1=X$, and $X_2=X^2$, Y turns out to be a quadratic function: $Y=a_0+a_1X+a_2X^2$.

Readers are referred to studies by Tanaka (1973) and Yamaguchi *et al.* (1970), in which three (urban, intermediate, and rural) and four (as seen in Tables 1 and 2 of this text) groups, respectively, are used for four values of inbreeding coefficients: $f=0$ (unrelated), $f=1/64$ (2nd cousin), $f=$

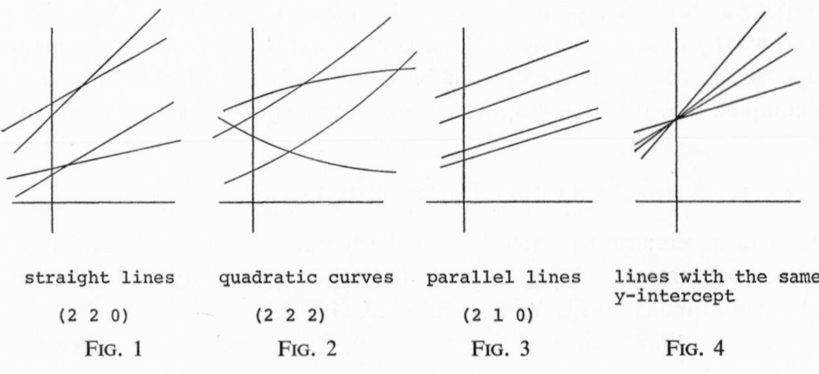

straight lines (2 2 0) FIG. 1

quadratic curves (2 2 2) FIG. 2

parallel lines (2 1 0) FIG. 3

lines with the same y-intercept FIG. 4

1/32 (1½ cousin), f=1/16 (cousin). Our program performs all plausible analyses by a single batch of input. Some of the analyses are illustrated in Figures 1, 2, 3, and 4. These figures show four different types to be fitted to the data consisting of four groups. A triplet of numbers is associated to indicate the model or the assumed situation. In Figure 1, four straight lines are fitted, and the coefficients to the quadratic term X^2 are all zero; thus in (2 2 0) the third entry is equal to zero. In Figure 3, the third entry of (2 1 0) is also zero, and, as the parallel lines are fitted:

$$
\begin{aligned}
Y^{(1)} &= a^{(1)} + a_1X,\\
Y^{(2)} &= a^{(2)} + a_1X,\\
Y^{(3)} &= a^{(3)} + a_1X,\\
Y^{(4)} &= a^{(4)} + a_1X,
\end{aligned}
$$

the coefficient to the linear term X is homogeneous for all of four groups; hence the second entry is 1. The triplet of numbers (1 2 0) in Figure 4 is obtained by interchanging the first and the second of Figure 3, showing that straight lines with the same y-intercept are fitted:

$$
\begin{aligned}
Y^{(1)} &= a_0 + a_1{}^{(1)}X,\\
Y^{(2)} &= a_0 + a_1{}^{(2)}X,\\
Y^{(3)} &= a_0 + a_1{}^{(3)}X,\\
Y^{(4)} &= a_0 + a_1{}^{(4)}X.
\end{aligned}
$$

In a triplet, the numbers 0, 1, and 2 indicate that the corresponding terms are nonexistent (0), existent and homogeneous (1), or existent and heterogeneous (2).

Of course there are other cases. The model (2 2 1) seems quite plausible, but it is hard to find an adequate nomenclature. The model (1 2 2) represents different curves sharing the same y-intercept, but this is hardly plausible. (2 0 0) represents fitting different constants, and (1 0 0), the same constant; a comparison of the outcomes of these two is called a test of homogeneity, and the usual method is a use of the χ^2 test. The totality of all plausible models forms a hierarchy, and we have considered the logics involved in the interpretation of outcomes of the analysis involving a hierarchy (Ito and Kudô, 1974, 1976). We are not repeating all the logics in interpretation here.

In addition to the logics we have developed, another notion is worth mentioning here: "Akaike Identification Criterion" (AIC). AIC was derived in a heuristic manner in order to determine how many unknown parameters are to be taken into a model. If the number of estimated parameters is equal to the number of observations (in a frequency data this number is that of figures in terms of percentage, and is not the number of individuals upon which the percentage figures are derived), the fit is usually perfect and no information is obtainable about the error. If the number of parameters is small, the model does not reflect the reality at all. AIC was derived to arrive at an adequate compromise (Akaike, 1974).

Although AIC was derived independently of Mallows's C_P statistic (Mallows, 1973), AIC happens to be a generalized version. A particular model is said to be adequate if the AIC value calculated from data under this model is smaller than the AIC values of any other plausible models.

The definition of the Akaike Identification Criterion is AIC=−2 [log (maximized likelihood)−number of estimated parameters]. The adequacy of AIC is yet to be examined in various situations, but it seems to have been proved useful in time series analysis. In our particular case, the values of AIC are quite concordant with the outcomes of our above-cited logic.

We present only one example: analyses of death rate within 10 years after birth from Yamaguchi *et al.* (1970), employing both logit as well as exponit models in Tables 1 and 2.

TABLE 1

	LOGIT Model	$P = 1/(1+e^Y)$
Year of birth	Y	Y
1929–35	$-1.59+1.05X-4.19X^2$	$-1.76+1.02X$
1936–40	$-1.70+1.05X-4.19X^2$	$-1.84+1.02X$
1941–45	$-1.68+1.05X-4.19X^2$	$-1.82+1.02X$
1946–50	$-2.35+1.05X-4.19X^2$	$-2.49+1.02X$
	$\chi^2=7.09$ d.f. $=10$	$\chi^2=9.95$ d.f. $=11$
	AIC = 4604.1	AIC = 4604.4

TABLE 2

	EXPONIT Model	$P = 1-e^{-Y}$
Year of birth	Y	Y
1929–35	$0.176+0.0982X-0.312X^2$	$0.165+0.0994X$
1936–40	$0.158+0.0982X-0.312X^2$	$0.147+0.0994X$
1941–45	$0.160+0.0982X-0.312X^2$	$0.150+0.0994X$
1946–50	$0.093+0.0982X-0.312X^2$	$0.082+0.0994X$
	$\chi^2=9.55$ d.f. $=10$	$\chi^2=11.27$ d.f. $=11$
	AIC = 4606.6	AIC = 4605.8

For technical reasons, X is a transformed variable from inbreeding coefficient F: $X=6.4F-0.2$; thus $X=-.2$ (unrelated), $-.2$ (2nd cousin), .0 (1½ cousin) and .2 (cousin). The minimum value of AIC is attained by the model (2 1 0): parallel line or (2 1 1): three quadratic lines, where only constant terms are heterogenous over these four groups according to year of birth. By the logic we have developed, we arrived at the same conclusion; i.e., (2 1 0) and (2 1 1) might well be adequate models.

In Tanaka's (1973) study, the groups represent the environmental differences: urban, intermediate, and rural; in Yamaguchi *et al.*'s (1970) study, they represent the year of birth, and reflect a large variation among the periods before, during, and after World War II. All the analyses consistently show that the models (2 1 0) or (2 1 1) fit the data quite well. This might well indicate that environmental variations are reflected in constant terms, while genetic factors are represented in the linear term, and also in the quadratic term, if it exists, and they remain the same in spite of the environmental changes.

It is also noteworthy that when we convert the values of Y to expected mortalities, we cannot find any substantial difference between exponit and logit models. Nevertheless, we are naturally led to ask, "Which model is more adequate?"

Comparision of Logit and Exponit Models

The exponit model was introduced in the field of population genetics by Morton, Crow, and Muller (1956). This model was derived assuming certain chance mechanisms behind the data, and it is related to the important notion of lethal equivalents per gamate. Therefore we ought to be very careful in employing a model other than the exponit model in the study of inbreeding effects.

We cannot, however, deny the advantages of the logit model over the exponit model. First of all, the logit model is very easy in numerical calculations. When the exponit model is used, special care must be taken in choosing the initial values before starting iterations, in order to arrive at the maximum likelihood estimate; in case of the logit model, the initial values are all taken as 0.1 for experimental reasons, and the iterations never fail to converge in hundreds of computations.

In addition to this, there are mathematically nice properties, including the fact that the logit model admits sufficient statistics. The most remarkable advantage was originally pointed out by K. P. Ito and used in Ito and Kudô (1976); it is demonstrated in the following example:

Suppose a pair of binary response variables (U, V), and assume the logit model is valid:

$$P_1 = P_r(U=1) = e^{Y_1}/(1+e^{Y_1}),\ 1-P_1 = P_r(U=0) = 1/(1+e^{Y_1})$$
$$P_2 = P(V_r=1) = e^{Y_2}/(1+e^{Y_2}),\ 1-P_2 = P_r(V=0) = 1/(1+e^{Y_2})$$

where

$$Y_1 = a_1{}^1X_1 + \ldots + a_n{}^1X_n$$
$$Y_2 = a_1{}^2X_1 + \ldots + a_n{}^2X_n\,.$$

We have four possible combinations of the values of (U, V):

(1 1)	(1 0)	U = 1
(0 1)	(0 0)	U = 0
$V=1$	$V=0$	

and repeated observations on (U, V) form an ordinary 2×2 contingency table:

N_{11}	N_{12}	$N_{1\cdot}$
N_{21}	N_{22}	$N_{2\cdot}$
$N_{\cdot 1}$	$N_{\cdot 2}$	$N_{\cdot\cdot}$

In forming such a contingency table, we are interested in the dependence or association between U and V, and if we assume the logit model in the combination of (U, V), we have to introduce a new function:

$$Y_3 = a_1{}^3X_1 + \ldots + a_n{}^3X_n\,.$$

The joint probabilities are expressed, after some calculations, in the following form:

e^{Y_3}/Z	e^{Y_1}/Z	$e^{Y_1}/(1+e^{Y_4}) = P_1$
e^{Y_2}/Z	$1/Z$	$1/(1+e^{Y_1}) = 1-P_2$
$e/(1\ {}^{Y_2}+ e^{Y_2}),$ $= P_2$	$1/(1+e^{Y_2})$ $=1-P_2$	

where

$$Z = 1 + e^{Y_1} + e^{Y_2} + e^{Y_3}\,.$$

In case U and V are independent, or there is no association between them, we can argue that $Y_3 = Y_2 + Y_1$. Thus the association or dependence between U and V can be assessed by the function

$$Y_3 - (Y_1 + Y_2) = (a_1{}^3 - (a_1{}^1 + a_1{}^2))X_1 + \dots + (v_n{}^3 - (a_n{}^1 + a_n{}^2))X_n.$$

These coefficients to $X_1, \dots, X_n$ are expected to be estimable in our empiric risk data. This is the reason why we anticipate that the logit model will be more advantageous than the linear and/or exponit models, which do not possess the property demonstrated above.

Acknowledgement
The author is very much grateful to Dr. Koichi P. Ito for detailed discussion of the content of this paper.

REFERENCES

Akaike, H. 1974. A new look at the statistical model identification. *IEEE Trans. on Automat. Contr.* **19**(6): 716–723.

Arikawa, S. 1975. Document retrieval using MIR-RF system. Proc. *Intl. Computer Symposium* vol. 2, 380–389.

Arikawa, S., and Kitagawa, T. 1975. *Multi-stage information retrieval system based upon researcher file*. Research Report No. 51, Research Institute of Fundamental Information Science, Kyushu Univ., Fukuoka, Japan.

Freire-Maia, Newton. 1973. Empiric risks in genetic counseling. *Soc. Biol.* **17**(3): 207–212.

Herndon, C. N. 1962. Empiric risks. *In* Burdette, W. J. (Ed.), *Methodology in human genetics*, pp. 144–155. Holden-Day, San Francisco, U.S.A.

Ito, P. K., and Kudô, A. 1975. Some logical issues in interpreting multivariate data by means of regression analysis. *In* Corsten, L. C. A., and Postelnicu, T. (Eds.), *Proceedings of the 8th international biometric conference*, pp. 85–101, Editura Academiei Republicii Socialiste Romania, Constanta, Romania.

Ito, P. K., and Kudô, A. 1976. A logistic regression analysis of bivariate binary data: A method of assessment for associations between a pair of binary responses. *J. Jap. Stat. Soc.* **6** (2): 5–15.

Kudô, A. 1962. A method for calculating the inbreeding coefficient. *Am. J. Hum. Genet.* **14**(14): 426–432.

Kudô, A., and Ito, P. K. 1975. Certain statistical methods in the analysis of inbreeding effect on mortality. *In* Corsten, L. C. A., and Postelnicu, T. (Eds.), *Proceedings of the 8th international biometric conference*, pp. 325–336. Editura Academiei Republicii Socialiste Romania, Constanta, Romania.

Mallows, C. L. 1973. Some comments on Cp. *Technometrics* **15**(4): 661–675.

Maruyama, T., and Yasuda, N. 1970. Use of graph theory in computation of inbreeding and kinship coefficients. *Biometrics* **26**(2): 209–219.

Morton, N. E., Crow, J. F., and Muller, H. J. 1956. An estimate of the mutational damage in man from the data on consanguineous marriages. *Proc. Natl. Acad. Sci.* (U.S.A.) **42**: 885–863.

Tanaka, K. 1973. Genetic studies on inbreeding in some Japanese populations. XI. Effects of inbreeding on mortality in Shizuoka. *Jap. J. Hum. Genet.* **17**(4): 319–331.

Yamaguchi, M. *et al.* 1970. Effects of inbreeding on mortality in Fukuoka population. *Am. J. Hum. Genet.* **22**(2): 145–159.

DISCUSSION 1

Estimating Empiric Risks in Practice

Charles Smith

Empiric risks are estimates of the recurrence risk of a disease in affected families. They are derived from observed data and do not depend on any model or genetic hypothesis. Much of their appeal lies in their apparently simple, practical, empiric nature. Their disadvantages lie in that they apply to the average family and do not allow extension to specific families, they deal with the particular population (and period) in which the data were collected, and they do not provide any understanding or generality in estimating recurrence risks. Another problem often ignored is that the risks may be difficult to estimate in practice. I would like to illustrate some of the problems in estimating empiric risks from some data on diabetes collected in Edinburgh, Scotland, during 1966–68. Data were available on 1367 diabetic probands and on some 25,000 relatives of different kinds (Falconer, Duncan, and Smith, 1971).

In practice there may be changes in the frequency of diabetes with time, due to changes in environment and nutrition or to changes in the levels of diagnosis and screening. There is also differential mortality among diabetics, the more severe cases having higher mortality, and so the sample of probands may not be an unbiassed one. There is also differential mortality of diabetics compared with non-diabetics so that the population prevalence, and the frequency among (living?) relatives, may be reduced. An attempt was made to adjust for these factors and to estimate the 'potential prevalence'—the prevalence expected if there was no differential mortality and detection levels remained at their current rate. The observed and estimated potential population prevalences in Edinburgh were:

	% with diabetes by age			
Population prevalence	25	45	65	85
Observed	0.2	0.5	1.7	1.4
Estimated potential	0.3	0.9	3.8	9.2

Agricultural Research Council, Animal Breeding Research Organisation, Edinburgh, Scotland.

The potential prevalence was very much higher than the observed prevalence, showing that even the population risks depend greatly on the basis used for estimating them.

For a disease with a variable age at onset, estimation of empiric risks is much more complex than for conditions manifest at birth or early in life. The age at onset of the proband and affected relatives must be taken into account and the risks of manifesting the disease by successive ages, as well as the total risk, will usually be required. In addition the family history of the disease may increase with time, as further family members become affected, and so empiric risks calculated from data with the *current* family history will tend to underestimate the actual risk (Darlow, Smith, and Duncan, 1973). To assess the importance of changes in family history, risks were estimated for families with the required family history (say with the proband and one sib affected) and for families with *at least* the required family history (with the proband, one affected sib, and zero, one, or more other affected relatives). The latter risks were on average about 1.3 times the former risks, again showing that the basis for estimating the empiric risks is important.

With such a large body of data (25,000 relatives) it would have seemed that quite accurate estimates of empiric risk would be obtained. However, this was not so because it was always necesssary to subdivide the data into various subgroups; for example, by kind and degree of genetic relationship to the proband (i.e., into parents, sibs, uncles-aunts, nephews-nieces, cousins, and children). There are also differences in population frequency, and in risks, due to sex. Moreover the ages at onset of the proband and of any affected relatives are important in assigning risks to the rest of the family, and further subdivisions are necessary to derive empiric risks for different proband–affected relative onset combinations. These and other causes of partition fragment the data into smaller and smaller portions so that the final empiric risks derived may have quite a high sampling variance (since the trait is all or none, diseased or affected) and may be unreliable.

I would refer you to the paper (Darlow *et al.*, 1973) for the actual empiric risk estimates we derived. My main objective here has been to highlight some of the difficulties in deriving and applying empiric risk estimates in practice.

REFERENCES

Darlow, J. M., Smith, C., and Duncan, L. J. P. 1973. A statistical and genetical study of diabetes. III, Empiric risks to relatives. *Ann. Hum. Genet.* **37**: 157–174.

Falconer, D. S., Duncan, L. J. P., and Smith, C. 1971. A statistical and genetical study of diabetes. I. Prevalence and morbidity. *Ann. Hum. Genet.* **34**: 347–369.

DISCUSSION 2

A Few Comments on Dr. Kudô's Paper

Koichi Ito

I have been associated with Dr. Kudô for some years in connection with the analysis of biometric data, and would like to elaborate some of the ideas presented in the second part of his paper from the standpoint of theoretical statistics.

In the second part of his paper Dr. Kudô dealt with the analysis of frequency data which is to be used to estimate empiric risks of common diseases. I am rather surprised to note that empiric risk is rather ambiguously defined. Empiric risk, as it is understood, is the probability of a certain event occurring estimated on the basis of previous knowledge and empirical observations rather than calculated on the basis of a certain genetic theory. The probability that an individual will succumb to a disease is usually affected by many factors, genetic and environmental. When the probability is to be estimated on the basis of statistical data, use must be made of regression analysis to interpret the given data.

Given a set or sets of data which are to be interpreted by means of regression analysis, we shall fit linear regression models to the data, based on a given set of independent variables and assuming a given form of relationship. In our joint papers (Ito and Kudô, 1975; 1976; Kudô and Ito, 1975), Dr. Kudô and I proposed to carry out a simultaneous analysis of all linear regression models of given form that are feasible under the circumstances where the data were collected and organized, and determine an adequate model, if any, from among the set of models, keeping in mind hierarchical relations among them.

The recent advances in computer technology enable us to perform a large number of analyses at the same time. We feel that this procedure of determining an adequate model in regression analysis will be particularly useful in the analysis of empiric risk data, where it is not clear which of many factors, genetic and environmental, are important and how they influence the risk. We also expect that this approach to the analysis of empiric risk data may shed some light on the question of goodness of fit of a model to the data

---

Nanzan University, Nagoya, Japan.

together with that of interactions between factors, which were raised in previous articles.

REFERENCES

Ito, K., and Kudô, A. 1975. Some logical issues in interpreting multivariate data by means of regression analysis. *In* Corsten, L. C. A., and Postelnicu, T. (Eds.), *Proceedings of the 8th international biometric conference*, pp. 85–101, Editura Academiei Republicii: Socialiste Romania, Constanta, Romania.

Ito, K., and Kudô, A. 1976. A logistic regression analysis of bivariate binary data: a method of assessing the association between a pair of binary responses, To appear in the Journal of Japan Statistical Society.

Kudô, A., and Ito, K. 1975. Certain statistical methods in the analysis of the effect of inbreeding on mortality. *In* Corsten, L. C. A., and Postelnicu, T. (Eds.) *Proceedings of the 8th international biometric conference*, pp. 325–336, Editura Academiei Republicii Socialiste Romania, Constanta, Romania.

Malformations in Monozygotic Twins: A Possible Example of Environmental Influence on the Developmental Genetic Clock

Ntinos C. Myrianthopoulos and Michael Melnick

Introduction

In this report we shall describe our attempts to gain some insight into the problem of gene-environment interaction through analysis of congenital malformations which occurred in twins born in the Collaborative Perinatal Project.

The Collaborative Perinatal Project is a cooperative endeavor, involving 12 institutions throughout the United States and the National Institute of Neurological and Communicative Disorders and Stroke of the National Institutes of Health, to observe and study events which affect the parents before and during pregnancy and to relate them to the outcome of pregnancy. To this end, about 56,000 pregnant women have been followed from the first months of their pregnancy through labor and delivery, and the children born to Project mothers are being followed to the seventh year of life. The Project population is about 45 percent White, 47 percent Negro, 7 percent Puerto Rican, and the rest a variety of other ethnic groups. The collection of information, medical examinations, and laboratory tests have been done in uniform fashion and according to preestablished protocol.

Twin pregnancies, of course, constitute only a small fraction of all pregnancies, and even in such a sizeable population as that of the Collaborative Perinatal Project, the number of twins available for study of congenital malformations would not be as large as one would have desired. The advantages, however, of prospective selection, nearly complete ascertainment, frequent examinations in accordance with a standardized protocol,

---

National Institute of Neurological and Communicative Disorders and Stroke, National Institutes of Health, Bethesda, Maryland, and Department of Oral-Facial Genetics, Indiana University School of Dentistry, Indianapolis, Indiana, U.S.A.

and assessment of malformations with high accuracy makes this a desirable twin population to study.

Criteria, Definitions, and Materials

The criteria for selection and definitions of congenital malformations have been described in detail in previous reports on malformations in singletons (Myrianthopoulos and Chung, 1974) and in twins (Myrianthopoulos, 1975). Briefly, a congenital malformation is defined as a gross physical or anatomic developmental anomaly which was present at birth or was detected during the first year of life. Malformations were divided into major and minor with some degree of arbitrariness: a malformation is considered major if it affects the individual adversely by causing increased mortality and morbidity. Otherwise it is considered minor.

The epidemiologic characteristics of twins born in the Collaborative Perinatal Project were described in a previous publication (Myrianthopoulos, 1970). To summarize, 615 pairs of twins were born among 56,249 pregnancies with known outcomes, or 1 in 91.5 births. Among Whites there were 259 twin births in 25,991 pregnancies, or 1 in 100.3 births; among Negroes there were 331 twin births in 26,080 pregnancies, or 1 in 78.8 births; and among the Other group, consisting mostly of Puerto Ricans, there were 25 twin births in 4,178 pregnancies, or 1 in 167.1 births.

The zygosity of 508 pairs of twins was established by comparison of sex, nine blood type systems (ABO, MNS, Rh, P, Kell, Lewis, Lutheran, Duffy, and Kidd), and gross and microscopic examination of the placenta. In 118 pairs the zygosity could not be determined. In some of these pairs one or both twins died early, before zygosity tests could be done, and placental examinations were not available or were inconclusive. Some were lost to the Project either because they were born outside a Project hospital or because their families withdrew their cooperation; in a few, the sex of one or both twins could not be determined.

Among White twins, 34.6 percent were monozygotic (MZ) and 65.4 percent dizygotic (DZ); among Negro twins 28.8 percent were MZ and 71.2 percent DZ; and among twins in the Other group, 60.0 percent were MZ and 40.0 percent DZ.

Included in this study are 1,197 twin individuals for whom information about the presence or absence of malformations was available. Their distribution by zygosity and completeness of pairs is shown in Table 1. This

TABLE 1. Twins at risk for malformations.

	Complete pairs	Incomplete pairs	Individuals
Monozygotic	187	1	375
Dizygotic	308	1	617
Zygosity undetermined	87	31	205
Total	582	33	1197

number includes 115 fetal and neonatal deaths for whom clinical and autopsy findings were available. Pairs were considered complete if information concerning malformations was available for both members of a pair, whether the twins were alive or dead. As is evident from Table 1, most of the incomplete pairs were in the zygosity undetermined (ZU) category.

Also included in this count is a pair of stillborn thoracopagus monozygotic female twins with multiple cardiovascular, alimentary, and other malformations. Because of the rarity and uniqueness of conjoined twinning, and the difficulty in ascribing the overall malformation as well as the specific malformations to one or the other twin, this pair was excluded from the calculation of malformation frequencies. It is used, however, in subsequent special analyses.

Malformations in Twins and Singletons

Table 2 shows the distribution of malformations in twins by zygosity. The last column gives the distribution of malformations in singletons from the same population for comparison. Numbers in parentheses represent frequencies of multiple malformations and individuals with multiple malformations; frequencies for single malformations are obtained by simple subtraction. Among 1,195 twin individuals for whom information about malformations was available, 219 or 18.33 percent were born with malformations—179 or 14.98 percent with single and 40 or 3.35 percent with multiple malformations. The total number of malformations was 294, of which 115 were multiple and were counted as many times as they occurred in an individual. Among malformed twins, 18.26 percent had more than one malformation, and 39.12 percent of malformations were associated with some other malformation.

Table 2 also shows that the frequency of malformations and malformed individuals is higher in twins than in singletons. Among 53,257 single deliveries in the Collaborative Perinatal Project, 8,288 or 15.56 percent

TABLE 2. Distribution of malformations in twins by zygosity, and in singletons (numbers in parentheses are multiple malformations).

	Twins				Singletons
	Monozygotic	Dizygotic	Zygosity undetermined	Total	
Total number of malformations	119 (44)	112 (36)	63 (35)	294 (115)	10,480 (3,574)
Total number of malformed cases	90 (15)	91 (15)	38 (10)	219 (40)	8,288 (1,382)
Total number of individuals	373	617	205	1195	53,257
Frequency (mean number) of malformations	0.319	0.181	0.307	0.246	0.197
Frequency of malformed cases (%)	24.13 (4.02)	14.75 (2.43)	18.54 (4.88)	18.33 (3.35)	15.56 (2.59)
Frequency of multiple malformations among all malformations (%)	36.97	32.14	55.56	39.12	34.10
Frequency of multiply malformed cases among all malformed cases (%)	16.67	16.48	26.32	18.26	16.67

were born with malformations—6,906 or 12.97 percent with single and 1,382 or 2.59 percent with multiple malformations. The increase of malformed twins over singletons is significant ($X_1^2=6.76$). Among malformed singletons, 16.67 percent had more than one malformation, and 34.10 percent of malformations were associated with some other malformation. The increase, however, of multiple malformations and multiple malformed individuals in twins over singletons is not significant.

These are among the highest malformation rates reported for twins and singletons. The high frequency of malformations could easily be explained on the basis of the period of time through which the malformations were observed and the conditions which made almost complete ascertainment possible.

It becomes evident, from closer inspection of Table 2, that the difference is entirely accounted for by an increase of malformations in MZ twins which is highly significant ($X_1^2=20.62$). DZ twins, if anything, show a slight decrease in frequency of malformations compared to singletons, but this is not significant. ZU twins show a frequency intermediate between those of MZ and DZ twins and similar to the overall twin malformation frequency. This is understandable since ZU twins comprise a mixture of MZ and DZ like-sexed twins. The increase in frequency of malformations in MZ twins holds true for both major and minor malformations. It is interesting that the slight decrease in malformation frequency of DZ twins observed in our data was also found by Hay and Wehrung (1970) in unlike-sexed twins for the malformations which they investigated.

Genetic analysis of twin data centers around comparisons of concordance in MZ and DZ twins. These provide a very useful screening technique for dealing with conditions in which a genetic component is suspected, and for obtaining some measure of the relative importance of genetic and environmental factors. The underlying principle is simple: the members of a pair of MZ twins are genetically identical and permit observations of the effects of differing environments on the same genotype, while the members of a pair of DZ twins are genetically different and permit studies of the effects of similar environment on different genotypes. Thus, twin research is not so much a tool for genetic analysis as a means for testing hypotheses about enviromental effects.

The practical application of this seemingly simple and elegant concept, however, is appreciably marred by several well-known experimental limitations and methodologic pitfalls (Allen, 1965), among which sampling bias and insufficient numbers must be placed at the top of the list. In the case of congenital malformations, the twin method has the additional disadvantage of confusing shared genotype with shared egg cytoplasm.

To overcome some of these pitfalls and limitations, some workers advocate the use of the proband concordance rates method of analysis, which is an application of the liability or threshold model for multifactorial inheritance (Falconer, 1965). This method uses concordance rates and incidences to provide estimates of correlation among twins in liability or threshold for a condition (Bulmer, 1970; Smith, 1974). The model, however, is not altogether satisfactory, for it is based on a certain amount of circular reasoning and on assumptions which in some cases are not tenable (Bulmer, 1970; Hrubec and Allen, 1975). Furthermore, it gives no insight into the nature of environmental factors or the gene-environment interaction involved in the production of the condition.

In congenital malformations this is a crucial point. After all, only a handful of malformations can definitely be attributed to specific environmental stresses, such as thalidomide ingestion and rubella infection; a few malformations such as aqueductal stenosis and polycystic kidney are known to be inherited; some malformations and malformation syndromes have been shown to be due to chromosomal aberrations. But the vast majority of malformations is of unknown etiology, presumably due to interaction of genetic and and environmental factors. The relative role of these factors and their mode of interaction are unknown.

Rather than deal in generalities again, we have chosen to use the twin data to investigate a specific environmental variable, the type of placenta, and its role in the production of malformations in man.

The Role of the Placenta

We have already seen that the frequency of malformations and malformed individuals is significantly higher in MZ than in DZ twins, and that the latter have a malformation frequency equal to that of singletons. This observation is not new but is, nonetheless, puzzling and still unexplained. It is tempting to speculate that a common mechanism may be responsible for both MZ twinning and congenital malformations, but evidence for this is lacking in man. In any case, the observation may in itself constitute a valuable clue about the occurrence of malformations whose etiology is unknown, and this is worth exploring.

The probability of occurrence of genetic malformations should be equal in MZ and DZ twins. Therefore, the excess malformations in MZ twins must be due to environmental factors, either acting directly on the developing embryo or interacting with the genetic determinants for normal embryonic development.

The importance of the human placenta in such processes is obvious. In twins, the placenta is a particularly good candidate for investigation. It is a physical and physiological link between mother and child; and it exhibits variations with regard to membrane type, size, shape, and circulation which may be important in themselves or may affect the nutrition of the embryo or the transport of drugs, toxins, and infectious agents which are important in the production of malformations.

The placentation of DZ twins is the same as that of singletons—each DZ twin individual is surrounded by a separate amnion and a separate chorion. MZ twins, however, can be either monochorionic (MC) or dichorionic (DC) depending on the time of separation of the cell mass which results in the two embryos. A small proportion of MZ twins also has a single amnion. In our series of 615 pairs, 9 or 1.5 percent were monoamniotic-monochorionic (MA-MC). Since DZ twins have the same placentation and the same malformation rate as singletons, we will confine our attention to differences in the placentation of MZ twins.

Several studies have shown that about two-thirds of MZ twins are MC and one-third are DC (see Bulmer, 1970, p. 31). Our data, shown in Table 3, agree with these figures. Among the 188 MZ pairs, 117 were MC and 56 DC, giving a ratio of 2.09:1. In 15 pairs the placentation could not be determined either because the placental material was unsuitable for examination or because the examination was not decisive.

Now, if we hypothesize that the excess malformations are environmentally

TABLE 3. Distribution of all MZ pairs and pairs with malformations, by placental type.

Placenta	All pairs	Pairs with malformations	% pairs with malformations
MC	117	42	35.90
DC	56	17	30.36
Unk.	15	7	46.67
Total	188	66	35.11
MC/DC ratio	2.09:1	2.47:1	

induced and due to influences of placental type or circulation, then we would expect higher proportions of malformations in MC than in DC twins. Our data, as shown in Table 3, do not support this hypothesis. The distribution by placental type of pairs with malformations is not significantly different from that of all pairs, and the frequency of MC pairs with malformations is not significantly different from that of DC pairs. The same is true when twins are considered as individuals rather than in pairs (Table 4). MC and DC MZ twins have frequencies of malformations in proportion to their distribution in the general population.

Concordance studies with regard to placental type should be illuminating, but with comparisons restricted to MZ pairs only, the available small numbers become even smaller. The findings, therefore, must be interpreted with caution.

Among the 66 pairs with one or both members malformed, the placental type was known in 59 pairs, 42 MC and 17 DC; in seven pairs the placental type was not known. Under the previously mentioned hypothesis we would expect significantly higher concordance among MC than among DC twins. It is evident from Table 5 that this is not the case. If anything, the concordance rate is higher among DC than among MC twins. This finding may be due to sampling error because of the small number of DC pairs. The binomial probability of obtaining this placental distribution of concor-

TABLE 4. Distribution of malformed individuals in MZ pairs with malformations.

Placenta	Pairs×2	Malformed individuals	% malformed individuals
MC	84	58	69.05
DC	34	24	70.59
Unk.	14	10	71.43
Total	132	92	69.70

TABLE 5. Concordance and discordance of MC and DC MZ twins in malformed sample.

Placenta	Conc.	Disc.	Concordance rate
MC	11	31	0.26
DC	10	7	0.59
Unk.	2	5	0.26

$\chi_1^2=4.29$, $p<0.05$

TABLE 6. Malformations in concordant MZ twins.

	Placenta	Twin A	Twin B
1	DC	Undescended testis	Undescended testis
2	MC	Macrocephaly	Hydrocephaly
3	DC	Metatarsus adductus; undescended testis	Metatarsus adductus
4	MC	Metatarsus adductus	Metatarsus adductus
5	DC	Metatarsus adductus	Metatarsus adductus
6	DC	Clinodactlyly	Clinodactyly
7	DC	Preauricular sinus	Ventricular septal defect
8	DC	Cystic kidney	Cardiac enlargement
9	MC	Focal malformation of bile duct; cystic kidney	Focal malformation of bile duct
10	MC	Hyperflexibility of knee joints	Anencephaly; cleft lip and palate; cor triloculare; absence of gall bladder; vertebral abnormality
11	DC	Polydactyly	Polydactyly
12	MC	Conjoined thoracopagus twins with fused hearts, livers, common umbilical cord and single placenta	
13	MC	Tracheoesophageal fistula	Cardiac enlargement; strawberry hemangioma
14	MC	Polydactyly	Polydactyly
15	DC	Deformed ear pinna	Deformed ear pinna
16	Unk.	Metatarsus adductus; inguinal hernia	Metatarsus adductus
17	MC	Metatarsus adductus	Metatarsus adductus
18	MC	Metatarsus adductus	Preauricular sinus
19	Unk.	Talipes equinovarus	Metatarsus adductus
20	DC	Deformed ear pinna; talipes calcaneovalgus	Deformed ear pinna; fibrous dysplasia of bone
21	DC	Pyloric stenosis; umbilical hernia; inguinal hernia	Pyloric stenosis; umbilical hernia; inguinal hernia
22	MC	Supernumerary nipples; café-au-lait spots	Supernumerary nipples; café-au-lait spots
23	MC	Preauricular skin tag	Preauricular skin tag

dant pairs under the 1: 1 hypothesis is 0.168. These data, again, lend no support to the hypothesis of placental effects.

Table 6 describes the malformations for which the 23 MZ pairs were concordant. Notice that not all of them were concordant for the same malformation. Sixteen pairs or 69.6 percent were concordant for at least one similar malformation and seven pairs or 30.4 percent were concordant for different malformations. Two pairs, Nos. 12 and 22, were MA-MC. The former is the pair of conjoined thoracopagus twins mentioned earlier. This pair has been described in detail elsewhere because of some interesting events in the history of the mother before and during pregnancy (Myrianthopoulos and Chung, 1975; Myrianthopoulos and Burdé, in press).

Some of these malformations are known to be genetic in origin (polydactyly, clinodactyly, supernumerary nipples, pyloric stenosis). Even when pairs with these genetic malformations are excluded (Table 7), the distribution of placental types does not appreciably change—nine pairs are MC and seven are DC. The binomial probability of obtaining this distribution under the 1: 1 hypothesis is 0.175.

These findings, though based on small numbers, provide fairly convincing evidence that the placenta and placental circulation *per se* do not contribute to the excess of malformations seen in MZ twins. And though they dash our expectations of gaining some insight into the problem through this important environmental variable, they provide, in a negative way, some clues on which to build a plausible hypothesis of gene-environment interaction in the causation of malformations.

TABLE 7. Placental type of concordant MZ twins.

Placenta	All pairs	Excluding pairs with genetic malformations*
MC	11	9
DC	10	7
Unk.	2	2

* Clinodactyly, #6; polydactyly, #11, 14; pyloric stenosis, #21; supernumerary nipples, #22.

A New Hypothesis

We propose that the excess of malformations in MZ twins is the result of a two-hit process: (1) the MZ twinning process which may occur anywhere from the pre-morula to the blastula stage disrupts the developmental genetic clock of the embryo; and (2) this disruption effects numerical and temporal biochemical disadvantages in the two resulting embryos and renders them susceptible to the action of subtle environmental agents.

The nature of genetic control of cellular spatial arrangement and differentiation has occupied the attention of embryologists and cell biologists for several decades. By 1971 Wolpert had proposed, and provided some evidence for, the hypothesis that spatial patterns of cellular differentiation may be established by a two-step process. First, the cells would fix their positions with respect to particular boundaries or regions in a way similar to a two- or three-dimensional geometric coordinate lattice. Having accomplished this, a given cell or group of cells would then interpret this positional information by selecting its next step in differentiation according to its genome and developmental history.

In 1973, Summerbell, Lewis, and Wolpert analyzed the development of the chick limb as an example of a growing organ. Their quantitative results demonstrated that there is a temporal order in the laying down of successive structures in the limb. They suggested that the positional information involved with this order might very well be related to the number of mitoses that have occurred. Thus, the behavior of regions of cells would depend not only on the three-dimensional patterns of space, but also on the fourth dimension of time.

Recently, Holliday and Pugh (1975) suggested a molecular basis for this developmental clock. Consider a hypothetical repeating sequence of DNA —say, CATATATG—at the end of which is an operator or promotor sequence. A modification enzyme binds to the first repeating sequence and modifies a particular base or bases. When this is complete, the site of action for the enzyme is now eight bases closer to the operator sequence. This process will be repeated, once per cell division, as many times as there are repeats of the sequence. At the end of the precisely determined number of divisions, the operator or promotor site is altered in the way that has been mentioned, and a developmental switch comes into operation. This mechanism suggests a most important role for the incredibly large amount of genomic repetitive DNA which is not transcribed. Holliday and Pugh also provided an alternative mechanism for counting cell divisions based on the methylation of palindromic controlling sequences. Whichever hypothesis one selects, all the offspring from a progenitor cell will reach the same stage of development after they have been through a given number of mitotic divisions. As the clone expands and each cell takes a specific position in space, the clock may initiate one or more events that eventually lead to specific differences in cell types within that clone.

What does this all mean vis-à-vis monozygotic twinning? Dichorionic monozygotic twins divide at or before the morula stage—i.e., prior to the fifth day. Diamniotic monochorionic MZ twins divide between the fifth and tenth days, and monoamniotic monochorionic MZ twins divide between the tenth and fourteenth days. Regardless of the number of cells present at division, if the division was relatively even, then for any specific point in early embryologicc time MZ twin embryos will be one mitotic step behind their normal singleton or DZ counterparts. This raises at least two interesting possibilities: (1) the embryo with H number of cells will, after dividing, have a developmental clock "set" for H, and this clock is "reset" to reflect the ½H cell number in each of the two twin embryos; or (2) the ½H cells are not "reset" and continue to reflect a developmental stage one mitotic step ahead of their actual number. Given the first possibility, the developmental time lag would probably be short, permitting quick restoration of the correct developmental clock stage. Thus, the process of MZ twinning would provide no more than a momentary disadvantage, hardly the stuff that malformations are made of.

If the developmental clock which controls the biochemical specificity of the cell surface is not reset, so to speak, then at least two more possibilities must be considered: (1) the nature of the cell surface antigens dictates the migration time of the cell mass and migration begins before sufficient number of cells have accrued leading to a cell number abberration; or (2) migration has little or nothing to do with the cell surface; instead it wholly depends on a requisite cell number. Thus, with the clock still running, the length of time available for spatial organization at the site of the future organ vis-à-vis the specific cell surface protein would possibly be reduced, resulting in some disorganization of the cell mass. This would also hold true for temporally sensitive induction.

The current embryologic and teratologic knowledge would tend to support the "cell surface dependent" possibility. Specific receptor sites on the surfaces or embryonic cells are thought to be involved in controlling cellular migration and adhesiveness (Oppenheimer *et al.*, 1969; Friberg *et al.*, 1971; Moscona, 1971). Neri *et al.*, (1975) have shown that only the migratory population of sea urchin embryonic cells are agglutinable with concanavalin A and exhibit concanavalin A-induced capping of receptor sites. Nonmigratory embryonic cell types do not exhibit these phenomena. Teratologic investigations by Poswillo (1974) into the pathogenesis of Treacher Collins syndrome indicated that the mechanism of malformation was early destruction of the neural crest cells of the facial and auditory primordia which migrate to the first and second branchial arches. That those structures affected in the face, jaw, and ear are not totally absent is due, in part, to the survival and migration of some neural crest cells. The work of Johnston and Pratt (1975) on the role of the neural crest in craniofacial development confirms these findings. Thus, it is clear that, in the absence of gene mutation, normal migration will commence and continue regardless of cell number, so long as the environment is not noxious.

It is conceivable that the disadvantages of cell number and, possibly, of biochemical timing which are brought about by the twinning process are in themselves sufficiently severe to increase significantly the malformation frequency in MZ twins. We consider it more likely, however, that the increase in malformations is due to the synergistic action of a disadvantaged embryo and to exposure to environmental agents that would be either non-teratogenic or only mildly teratogenic in DZ twins and in singletons who have not been subjected to the first hit. The list of such agents in our increasingly polluted world, both industrially and pharmacologically, is certainly on the rise. For example, Shields (1976) has shown that sporadic, environmentally-induced isolated cleft palate in Denmark has significantly increased during the years 1956–1970 as compared to 1941–1955. In addition, pharmaceuticals once thought safe are now known not to be so (Villumsen, 1970; Levy *et al.*, 1973; Janerich *et al.*, 1974; Milkkorrich and Van den Berg, 1974; Saxén, 1975).

The proposed hypothesis can be tested by a variety of experimental approaches. It is possible, for example, to study epidemiologically the frequency of drug intake, viral infections, febrile episodes, etc., during pregnancy of mothers of MZ twins in comparison to that of mothers of DZ twins and singletons. Such a study, using Collaborative Perinatal Project data, is under way. Another approach would be by a well-controlled teratologic study designed to demonstrate the synergistic relationship described above. One can induce MZ twinning in chicks and/or non-multiparous mammals and in one group introduce a mild teratogen early in embryogenesis. If the hypothesis is correct, then the frequency of malformations in that group should be significantly greater than the additive expectation derived from other groups of induced twins and singletons exposed to only a single treatment or no treatment at all. A third approach would be to attempt to trace the fate of the developmental clock by determining the length of time specific cell surface proteins are present during the formation of a given structure in induced twins vs. singletons (e.g., neural crest migration/organization and facial development).

Experiments of this sort not only may provide an explanation for the increased frequency of malformations in MZ twins but also would enhance our still lamentably meager understanding of the interaction between genes and environment in common disorders of man.

Acknowledgements

The Collaborative Study of Cerebral Palsy, Mental Retardation, and Other Neurological and Sensory Disorders of Infancy and Childhood is supported by the National Institute of Neurological and Communicative Disorders and Stroke. The following institutions participate: Boston Lying-In Hospital; Brown University; Charity Hospital, New Orleans; Children's Hospital of Buffalo; Children's Hospital of Philadelphia; Children's Medical Center, Boston; Columbia University; Johns Hopkins University; Medical College of Virginia; New York Medical College; Pennsylvania Hospital; University of Minnesota; University of Oregon; University of Tennessee and the Developmental Neurology Branch, NINCDS.

REFERENCES

Allen, G. 1965. Twin research: problems and prospects. *In* Steinberg, A. G., and Bearn, A. G. (Eds.), *Progress in medical genetics*, vol. 4, pp. 242–269. Grune & Stratton, New York, U.S.A.

Bulmer, M. G. 1970. *The biology of twinning in man*. Clarendon Press, Oxford, U.K.

Falconer, D. S. 1965. The heritability of liability to certain diseases estimated from the incidence among relatives. *Ann. Hum. Genet.* **29**: 51–76.

Friberg, S. J., Cochran, A. J., and Colub, S. H. 1971. Concanavalin A inhibits tumor cell migration. *Nature* (*New Biol.*) **232**: 121–122.

Hay, S., and Wehrung, D. A. 1970. Congenital malformations in twins. *Am. J. Hum. Genet.* **22**: 662–678.

Holliday, R., and Pugh, J. E. 1975. DNA modification mechanisms and gene activity during development. *Science* **187**: 226–232.

Hrubec, Z., and Allen, G. 1975. Methods and interpretation of twin concordance data. *Am. J. Hum. Genet.* **27**: 808–809.

Janerich, D. T., Piper, J. M., and Glebatis, D. M. 1974. Oral contraceptives and congenital limb-reduction defects. *N. Engl. J. Med.* **291**: 697–700.

Johnston, M. C., and Pratt, R. M. 1975. The neural crest in normal and abnormal craniofacial development. *In* Slavkin, H. C., and Greulick, R. C. (Eds.), *Extracellular matrix influences on gene expression*, pp. 773–777. Academic Press, New York, U.S.A.

Levy, E. P., Cohen, A., and Fraser, F. C. 1973. Hormone treatment during pregnancy and congenital heart defects. *Lancet* **1**: 611.

Milkkorrich, L., and Van den Berg, B. J. 1974. Effects of prenatal meprobamate and chlordiazepoxide hydrochloride in human embryonic and fetal development. *N. Engl. J. Med.* **29**: 1268–1271.

Moscona, A. A. 1971. Embryonic and neoplastic cell surfaces: Availability of receptors for concanavalin A and wheat germ agglutinin. *Science* **171**: 905–907.

Myrianthopoulos, N. C. 1970. An epidemiologic survey of twins in a large, prospectively studied population. *Am. J. Hum. Genet.* **22**: 611–629.

Myrianthopoulos, N. C. 1975. Congenital malformations in twins: epidemiologic survey. *Birth Defects: Orig. Art. Series*, Vol. XI, No. 8.

Myrianthopoulos, N. C., and Burdé, B. A case of conjoined twins. *Acta Genet. Med. Gemellol.* In press.

Myrianthopoulos, N. C., and Chung, C. S. 1974. Congenital malformations in singletons: Epidemiologic survey. *Birth Defects: Orig. Art. Series*, Vol. X, No. 11.

Neri, A., Roberson, M., Connolly, D. T., and Oppenheimer, S. B. 1975. Quantitative evaluation of concanavalin A receptor site distributions on the surfaces of specific populations of embryonic cells. *Nature* **258**: 342–344.

Oppenheimer, S. B., Edidin, M., Orr, C. W., and Roseman, S. 1969. An L-glutamine requirement for intercellular adhesion. *Proc. Nat. Acad. Sci. U.S. A.* **63**: 1395–1402.

Poswillo, D. 1974. Otomandibular deformity: pathogenesis as a guide to reconstruction. *J. Max-fac. Surg.* **2**: 64–72.

Saxén, I. 1975. Associations between oral clefts and drugs taken during pregnancy. *Int. J. Epidemiol.* **4**: 37–44.

Shields, E. D. 1976. Cleft palate in the Danish: A definition of etiologic heterogeneity and the developmental genetic implications. Ph.D. Thesis, Indiana University, U.S.A.

Smith, C. 1974. Concordance in twins: Methods and interpretation. *Am. J. Hum. Genet.* **26**: 454–466.

Summerbell, D., Lewis, J. H., and Wolpert, L. 1973. Positional information in chick limb morphogenesis. *Nature* **244**: 492–496.

Villumsen, A. L. 1970. *Environmental factors in congenital malformation: A prospective study of 9,006 human pregnancies*, pp. 30, 177–178. F.A.D.L.s Forlag, Copenhagen, Denmark.

Wolpert, L. 1971. Positional information and pattern formation. *Curr. Top. Dev. Biol.* **6**: 183–224.

DISCUSSION 1

Use of Twin Registers in the Study of Human Diseases

Eiji Inouye

Most of the past twin studies were based upon either cross-sectional data collected at one time or information obtained retrospectively. Obviously, the usefulness of cross-sectional data is limited in the study of chronic diseases. Retrospective information involves various sources of bias. In this connection, prospective studies will largely eliminate the limitations and bias sources. In this kind of study cohorts of twins are registered, and a collaborative study by Dr. Myrianthopoulos and his co-workers employed this kind of research design.

In conducting prospective studies there are many problems to be solved. Expenditures of funds, time, and labor are required, and we must decide which kinds of data, information, and sources of information should be kept in the register.

There is a twin register at our laboratory, whose research design is partly prospective. Subjects are candidates for admission to a junior high school, selected only for school performance and area of residence. Since 1948 a maximum of 22 pairs of twins has been admitted to the school every year, and at the admission, we are collaborating with the school in taking family and personal histories and performing zygosity diagnosis and medical checkups. We also give anthropometric, dermatoglyphic, biochemical, and other examinations, if the subjects, parents, and school teachers give consent.

In 1974, a female monozygotic twin student at the school was admitted to University of Tokyo Hospital with a diagnosis of systemic lupus erythematosus. Incidentally, a small amount of sera of this twin and her co-twin had been frozen and stored at our laboratory. The sera were taken three years before the onset of the disease in index twin and then separated from the blood sample used for zygosity diagnosis. We provided the hospital with the premorbid sera, and Drs. Horiuchi, Hashimoto, and others of the hospital found that DNA binding activity of the serum of index twin was about 20 percent higher than in normal controls, while that of the co-twin

Institute of Brain Research, University of Tokyo School of Medicine, Tokyo, Japan.

was in normal range. The co-twin has been well since the admission to the school, but after the onset of the disease in the index twin, the co-twin's DNA binding activity was found to be over 20 percent higher than normal value.

Another interesting finding in this twin pair is the response to Bacille Calmette Guélin (BCG) vaccination long before the onset of the disease. According to retrospective information obtained at the admission of the twins to the school, the index twin had always been tuberculin negative after BCG vaccination at primary school, while her co-twin became positive after vaccination. This suggests a possible acquired immune deficiency in the index twin, which may be relevant to the discordant manifestation of the disease in this twin pair.

The size of the twin cohort in this particular register is several hundred pairs, and it is difficult to obtain enough subjects to permit genetic analysis of complex etiological mechanisms involved, even if the disease is fairly common. In this connection, we started a pilot study in four districts of Japan, in which all multiple birth and stillbirth certificates are recorded with the permission of the officials in change. We are trying to link the data with other health records kept at various facilities. Privacy and confidentiality are most important in this kind of study, and we hope to establish double or triple safeguards by recording code numbers of the subjects instead of names, addresses, and other personal data. The record also includes sex, birth weight, and other items, but storing and retrieval of specimens and health check records taken on various occasions may be of crucial importance in the future. If a register is widely accepted and used as a kind of data bank, to which people deposit specimens and health records as their own, the present hazards in genetic-epidemiological and clinical studies on human diseases will be largely eliminated.

DISCUSSION 2

Comments on Genetic Load

Takeo Maruyama

I'd like to make two comments.

One is directly related to my subject which I discussed before in terms of genetic load, and the other is related to the general nature of the symposium.

I have shown data from *Drosophila* indicating that mildly detrimental mutations per genome or per chromosome occur at rates of ten to fifteen or even as high as thirty times those of lethal mutations. Now I should like to ask where this polygene comes from in terms of gene arrangement in the genome or otherwise. My first comment is going to be related to this, and the very high mutation rate for mildly detrimental genes seems to warrant two possible explanations.

The first possible explanation is that for each locus at which mutation produces lethals there are ten to twenty loci at which mutation produces detrimentals. Judd and his group (1972) at the University of Texas have demonstrated a one-to-one correspondence between the number of salivary bands and detectable complementation groups in the zeste to white region of the *Drosophila* X chromosome. Each detectable complementation group is, presumably, a structural gene since the mutations detected were either lethal, visible, or behavioral in nature; extrapolating, a figure of approximately six thousand structural genes per haploid genome is reached. The haploid genome, however, contains sufficient DNA for several times this number of genes. Mukai and Cockerham (1976) propose that mutations which occur in the DNA not coding for structural genes may have mildly detrimental effects and thus explain the observed ratio of deterimental to lethal mutations.

The alternative explanation is that virtually all mutations of interest occur in the structural genes; but, for a given locus, only a small proportion of mutants exhibit the extreme phenotype with the majority of mutants at the locus having little or no effect on the organism. From the genetic code, it is easily seen that a base pair substitution will result in a missense muta-

Department of Population Genetics, National Institute of Genetics, Mishima, Japan.

tion ten to twenty times as frequently as it will result in a nonsense mutation. Indeed, Whitfield, Martin, and Ames (1966) obtained a ten-to-one ratio of missense to nonsense mutations at the histidine locus of *Salmonella*. The altered polypeptide produced by the missense mutant is likely to retain some of the activity of the polypeptide coded for by the wild type from which the mutant was derived; thus the missense mutation may have only mild effects on the organism. I don't know whether the missense mutations found by Whitfield and his colleagues were mild or harmful (the nonsense mutants were lethal); but, in either case, the above argument remains valid and the experiment provides support for the hypothesis that the mutation rate per locus of mildly detrimental mutations is higher than that of lethal mutations.

I should like to make one more comment which bears on the essence of this symposium. That is; we have discussed mainly "diseases," but I should like to mention one example in which interaction between gene and environment has played a very important role in evolution in man, that is, brain evolution and our technology. I think the very nature of man is to have an advanced brain. And we may ask how this evolved. Some biologists think that is a result of interaction between an advanced brain and an advanced tool. To begin with, if man is to use a tool, a better brain would use it more efficiently, and an advanced brain can produce an advanced tool and use more wisely such a tool, and an advanced tool requires a still more advanced brain to use it, and so on. I think this interaction improves the brain in such a manner. It is very surprising that our brain evolved in capacity about three times in the last one million years, which is among the fastest evolution in a mammalian character as far as biologists know.

REFERENCES

Judd, B. H., Shen, M. W., and Kaufman, T. C. 1972. The antomy and function of a segment of the X chromosome of *Drosophila melanogaster*. *Genetics* **71**: 139–156.

Mukai, T., and Cockerham, C. 1976. Spontaneous mutation rates of isozyme genes in *Drosophila melanogaster*. *Proc. Nat. Acad. Sci. U. S.* (to appear).

Whitfield, H. J., Martin, R. G., and Ames, B. N. 1966. Classification of mutants in the C gene of the histidine operon. *Jour. Mol. Biol.* **21**: 335–355.

Concluding Remarks

N. E. Morton

I am substituting for Dr. Arno Motulsky, who was prevented from coming by influenza. He was greatly missed by everyone but perhaps especially by me, because Arno would have arrived with his ideas brilliantly conceived, deeply pondered, and neatly typed, whereas I have faced this meeting with unusual sobriety because of the very short notice for making these casual remarks. So, *gokuro sama deshita.*

In the opening session, Professor Inouye gave us a charge to look for tools of research on common diseases with the ultimate goal of prevention and therapy. The consensus has been that the polygenic model may be the best initial hypothesis because it provides a quantitative theory which incorporates multiple genetic and environmental factors into a single parameter describing recurrence risks.

Dr. Myrianthopoulos was among those who expressed concern that the model might be accepted too enthusiastically, so that effects of major loci and environmental agents might be missed. Clearly it is a challenge for genetic epidemiologists to devise good tests for such heterogeneity and to apply them critically to common diseases.

Diagnostic refinements have been and will probably continue to be more powerful than purely statistical analysis, which can, however, be an invaluable and objective aid. Mental retardation provides an example of this. A simple polygenic model predicts higher rates of affection for relatives of more severely retarded patients, but exactly the opposite is observed. The explanation is that mild cases have a large component due to polygenes and/or common environment, whereas severe cases are mostly sporadic or monogenic (sporadic cases include, of course, chromosome aberrations). Diagnostic resolution of heterogeneity gives a much better fit to segregation data and provides much more reliable and specific estimates of recurrence risks.

At each stage in our progressive understanding of the etiology of common diseases it is important to make results available to genetic counselling and to programs for prevention in high-risk groups. Empiric and genetic risks are becoming more reliable, but there is an opportunity for improvement of both.

Some common diseases with high levels of ascertainment lend themselves to surveillance against mutagens, teratogens, and carcinogens. Because of its relatively simple etiology, Down's syndrome is one obvious choice. Several studies have suggested interaction between maternal age and X-radiation. Furthermore, most cases are spontaneously aborted, so that incidence among liveborn is only a remnant of the incidence at conception. Boué suggests that the fraction recovered at birth may be influenced by medical treatment to prevent threatened abortion. Recent proof from chromosome polymorphism that some cases of Down's syndrome arise by paternal non-disjunction makes one wonder whether maternal age effects are not partly on fetal survival, and paternal factors (including irradiation) have been neglected. Similarly, an even larger proportion of triploids is aborted, and there is evidence that triploidy may be increased in women who recently abandoned or were irregular in the use of oral contraceptives. Probably other environmental agents predisposing to polyploidy will be identified.

In considering registers for affected liveborn, we must not forget the opportunities which spontaneous and induced abortions provide for genetic epidemiology and the detection of noxious environmental factors. I wonder if the admirable cytogenetics done by Dr. Awa and others in Hiroshima and Nagasaki might not profitably be extended to the richer populations provided by aborted chromosomal aberrations, which may offer more promise to detect mutation than a search for biochemical mutants, whose discrimination from parentage errors is more difficult and in a large proportion of cases impractical.

In conclusion I shall not attempt to review the symposium, which is much too complex for that. On behalf of the foreign visitors I would like to express our pleasure in attending this stimulating symposium. For the generosity of the Japan Medical Research Foundation, the superb site provided by the Toshi Medical Center, and the good company in meetings and receptions, our sincere thanks.

Participants

Masahiko ANDO
Heart Institute, Tokyo Women's Medical College, Tokyo, Japan
Masataka ARIMA
Division of Child Neurology, Tottori University School of Medicine, Yonago, Japan
Akio ASAKA
Institute of Brain Research, University of Tokyo School of Medicine, Tokyo, Japan
Isamu AWANO
Department of Medicine, Fukushima Medical School, Fukushima, Japan
Kazuo BABA
Department of Pediatrics, Faculty of Medicine, Nihon University, Tokyo, Japan
C. O. CARTER
MRC Clinical Genetic Unit, Institute of Child Health, London, Great Britain
Akira ENDO
Department of Hygiene and Preventive Medicine, Yamagata University School of Medicine, Yamagata, Japan
F. Clarke FRASER
Department of Biology and Pediatrics, McGill University, Station A Montreal, Quebec, Canada
Norio FUJIKI
Department of Genetics, Institute for Developmental Research, Aichi Prefectural Colony, Kasugai, Japan
Yoshishige FUJIKI
Department of Oral Radiology, Gifu College of Dentistry, Gifu, Japan
Yukio FUKUYAMA
Department of Pediatrics, Tokyo Women's Medical College, Tokyo, Japan

Toshiyuki FURUSHO
Department of Hygiene, Kagoshima University School of Medicine, Kagoshima, Japan

Jun-ichi FURUYAMA
Department of Genetics, Hyogo Medical College, Nishinomiya, Japan

Hideo HAMAGUCHI
Institute of Basic Medical Sciences, University of Tsukuba, Ibaraki, Japan

Yasushi HAYASHI
Research Institute of Environmental Medicine, Nagoya University, Nagoya, Japan

Yukimasa HAYASHI
Institute for Developmental Research, Aichi Prefectural Colony, Kasugai, Japan

Makoto HIGURASHI
Department of Maternal and Child Health, Faculty of Medicine, University of Tokyo, Japan

Kiyotake HIRAYAMA
Department of Pediatrics, Hospital of Ryukyu University, Naha, Japan

Munehiro HIRAYAMA
Department of Maternal and Child Health, Faculty of Medicine, University of Tokyo, Tokyo, Japan

Yoshihiko HORIUCHI
Department of Medicine and Physical Therapy, University of Tokyo School of Medicine, Tokyo, Japan

Kiyoshi HOSHINO
Research Institute of Environmental Medicine, Nagoya University, Nagoya, Japan

Kazuzo IINUMA
Department of Human Genetics, National Institute of Genetics, Mishima, Japan

Takayoshi IKEDA
First Department of Pathology, Nagasaki University School of Medicine, Nagasaki, Japan

Yoko IMAIZUMI
Population Quality Section, Institute of Population Problem, Ministry of Health and Welfare, Tokyo, Japan

Takashi IMAMURA
First Department of Medicine, Faculty of Medicine, Kyushu University, Fukuoka, Japan

Shigeko INOKUMA
Department of Medicine and Physical Therapy, University of Tokyo School of Medicine, Tokyo, Japan

Eiji INOUE
Professor, Institute of Brain Research, University of Tokyo School of Medicine, Tokyo, Japan

Katsuaki ITAKURA
Department of Pathology, Asahikawa Medical College, Asahikawa, Japan

Koichi ITO
Department of management, Faculty of Management, Nanzan University, Nagoya, Japan

Toshiharu JIMBO
Department of Obstetrics and Gynecology, University of Tokyo School of Medicine, Tokyo, Japan

Takeo JUJI
Blood Transfusion Service, University of Tokyo School of Medicine, Tokyo, Japan

Yoshiro KAMEYAMA
Research Institute of Environmental Medicine, Nagoya University, Nagoya, Japan

Hiroo KATO
Department of Epidemiology and Statistics, Radiation Effects Research Foundation, Hiroshima, Japan

Teruo KITAGAWA
Department of Pediatrics, Nihon University School of Medicine, Tokyo, Japan

Hideo KOGUCHI
Department of Oral Surgery, Faculty of Dentistry, Kyushu University, Fukuoka, Japan

Akira KOIZUMI
Department of Human Ecology, Faculty of Medicine, University of Tokyo, Tokyo, Japan

Kiyotaro KONDO
Department of Neurology, Brain Research Institute, Niigata University, Niigata, Japan

Kyoji KONDO
Department of Animal Sciences, Faculty of Agriculture, Nagoya University, Nagoya, Japan

Shunzo KONISHI
Department of Pediatrics, Yamaguchi University School of Medicine, Ube, Japan

Akio KUDO
Department of Mathematics, Faculty of Sciences, Kyushu University, Fukuoka, Japan

Soji KURITA
Outpatient Department, Aichi Cancer Center, Nagoya, Japan

Yoshigoro KUROIWA
Department of Neurology, Kyushu University School of Medicine, Fukuoka, Japan

Yoshikazu KUROKI
Department of Genetics, Kanagawa Children's Medical Center, Yokohama, Japan

Takeo MARUYAMA
Department of Population Genetics, National Institute of Genetics, Mishima, Japan

Ichiro MATSUI
Department of Genetics, Kanagawa Children's Medical Center, Yokohama, Japan

Ei MATSUNAGA
Department of Human Genetics, National Institute of Genetics, Mishima, Japan

Kazuya MIKAMO
Department of Biology, Asahikawa Medical College, Asahikawa, Japan

James, R. MILLER
Department of Medical Genetics, University of British Columbia, Vancouver, Canada

Goro MIMURA
Institute of Constitutional Medicine, Kumamoto University, Kumamoto, Japan

Seisho MIYAMOTO
First Department of Medicine, Faculty of Medicine, Kyushu University, Fukuoka, Japan

Akira MIZUTANI
Institute for Developmental Research, Aichi Prefectural Colony, Kasugai, Japan

Katsuhiko MORI
Heart Institute, Tokyo Women's Medical College, Tokyo, Japan

Iwao, M. MORIYAMA
Department of Epidemiology and Statistics, Radiation Effects Research Foundation, Hiroshima, Japan

Newton, E. MORTON
Population Genetics Laboratory, University of Hawaii at Manoa, Honolulu, Hawaii, U.S.A.

Arno, G. MOTULSKY
Division of Medical Genetics, Department of Medicine, University of Washington School of Medicine, Seattle, Washington, U.S.A.

Ujihiro MURAKAMI
Institute for Developmental Research, Aichi Prefectural Colony, Kasugai, Japan

Ntinos, C. MYRIANTHOPOULOS
Perinatal Research Branch, National Institute of Neurological and Communicative Disorders and Stroke, National Institute of Health, Bethesda, Maryland, U.S.A.

Setsuya NAITO
Department of Internal Medicine, Fukuoka University School of Medicine, Fukuoka, Japan

Yasuo NAKAGOME
Department of Human Genetics, National Institute of Genetics, Mishima, Japan

Hiroshi NAKAJIMA
Department of Biochemical Genetics, Medical Research Institute, Tokyo Medical and Dental University, Tokyo, Japan

Kazushige NAKAMURA
Department of Anatomy, Kobe University School of Medicine, Kobe, Japan

Minoru NAKATA
Department of Pedodontics, Tokyo Medical and Dental University School of Dentistry, Tokyo, Japan

Shin-ichiro NANKO
Institute of Brain Research, University of Tokyo School of Medicine, Tokyo, Japan

Hideo NISHIMURA
Department of Anatomy, Faculty of Medicine, Kyoto University, Kyoto, Japan

Hiroshi NOGAMI
Department of Embryology, Institute for Developmental Research, Aichi Prefectural Colony, Kasugai, Japan

Tatsuji NOMURA
Central Institute for Experimental Animals, Kawasaki, Japan

Yasuo OCHIAI
Institute for Developmental Research, Aichi Prefectural Colony, Kasugai, Japan

Zen-ichi OGITA
Department of Genetics, Osaka University School of Medicine, Osaka, Japan

Koji OHKURA
Department of Human Genetics, Medical Research Institute, Tokyo Medical and Dental University, Tokyo, Japan

Hidetsune OISHI
Department of Genetics, Institute for Developmental Research, Aichi Prefectural Colony, Kasugai, Japan

Michio OKAJIMA
Department of Forensic Medicine, Tokyo Medical and Dental University, Tokyo, Japan

Naomasa OKAMOTO
Research Institute for Nuclear Medicine and Biology, Hiroshima University, Hiroshima, Japan

Keiichi OMOTO
Department of Anthology, Faculty of Sciences, University of Tokyo, Tokyo, Japan

Kyung Sook PARK
Institute of Brain Research, University of Tokyo School of Medicine, Tokyo, Japan

Reiji SEMBA
Institute for Developmental Research, Aichi Prefectural Colony, Kasugai, Japan

Kohei SHIOTA
Department of Anatomy, Faculty of Medicine, Kyoto University, Kyoto, Japan

Ryujiro SHOJI
Institute for Developmental Research, Aichi Prefectural Colony, Kasugai, Japan

Charles SMITH
A. R. C. Animal Breeding Research Organization, Edinburgh, Scotland

Tsutomu SUGAHARA
Department of Experimental Radiology, Faculty of Medicine, Kyoto University, Kyoto, Japan

Yasuro SUGISHITA
Institute of Clinical Medicine, University of Tsukuba, Sakura-mura, Ibaragi, Japan

Yasuo SUGIURA
Department of Orthopaedic Surgery, Nagoya University School of Medicine, Nagoya, Japan

Masakuni SUZUKI
Department of Obstetrics and Gynecology, Tohoku University School of Medicine, Sendai, Japan

Atsuyoshi TAKAO
Heart Institute, Tokyo Women's Medical College, Tokyo, Japan

Takatada TAKASHIMA
Department of Pedeatrics, Nihon University School of Medicine, Tokyo, Japan

Yoh TAKEYA
Kyushu University Health Center, Fukuoka, Japan

Osamu TANAKA
Human Embryo Center for Teratological Studies, Faculty of Medicine, Kyoto University, Kyoto, Japan

Takashi TANIMURA
Department of Anatomy, Faculty of Medicine, Kyoto University, Kyoto, Japan

Katsumi TANAKA
Medical Research Institute, Tokyo Medical and Dental University, Tokyo, Japan

Hideo TASHIRO
Department of Oral Surgery, Faculty of Dentistry, Kyushu University, Fukuoka, Japan

Tamotsu TERAWAKI
Department of Pediatrics, Kagoshima University School of Medicine, Kagoshima, Japan

Akira TONOMURA
Department of Human Cytogenetics, Medical Research Institute, Tokyo Medical and Dental University, Tokyo, Japan

Kimiyoshi TSUJI
Blood and Tissue Typing Center, Tokai University School of Medicine, Isehara, Japan

Yoshiro WADA
Department of Pediatrics, Tohoku University School of Medicine, Sendai, Japan

Gen-ichi WATANABE
Department of Hygiene and Preventive Medicine, Niigata University School of Medicine, Niigata, Japan

Yukio YAMADA
National Institute of Animal Industry, Ministry of Agriculture and Forestry, Chiba, Japan

Masaya YAMAGUCHI
First Department of Medicine, Faculty of Medicine, Kyushu University, Fukuoka, Japan

Yukio YAMORI
Department of Pathology, Faculty of Medicine, Kyoto University, Kyoto, Japan

Mineo YASUDA
Department of Perinatology, Institute for Developmental Research, Aichi Prefectural Colony, Kasugai, Japan

Takato YOSHIDA
Department of Microbiology, Hamamatsu University School of Medicine, Hamamatsu, Japan

Toshiyuki YANASE
First Department of Medicine, Faculty of Medicine, Kyushu University, Kyushu, Japan

Executive Members of Japan Medical Research Foundation

(Adviser)

Zenko Suzuki	Ex-Minister of Health and Welfare

(Chairman)

Yoshizane Iwasa	Chairman, Fuji Bank

(President)

Masayoshi Yamamoto	Governor, Medical Care Facilities Finance Corporation

(Board of Trustees)

Masaaki Arai	President, Life Insurance Association of Japan
Nihachiro Hanamura	Executive Director, Federation of Economic Organizations
Yoshito Kobayashi, M. D.	President, Japanese Association of Medical Sciences
Yoshiyuki Koyama, M. D.	Director General, National Hospital Medical Center
Hiroshi Kumagaya, M. D.	Vice-President, Japanese Association of Medical Sciences
Shigeo Okinaka, M. D.	Professor Emeritus, University of Tokyo
Taro Takemi, M. D.	President, Japan Medical Association
Daizo Ushiba, M. D.	Professor, Keio University
Eiichi Wakamatsu, M. D.	President, Japan Public Health Association
Yuichi Yamamura, M. D.	Professor, Osaka University
Yawara Yoshitoshi, M. D.	President, Hamamatsu Medical College

(Inspectors)

Masao Kumazaki	President, Environmental Pollution Control Service Corporation
Yutaka Tateno, M. D.	Chairman, Medical Committee, Life Insurance Association of Japan